Physics of Quantum Electronics
Based on Lectures of Summer Schools
Volume 1

High Energy Lasers
and Their Applications

PHYSICS OF QUANTUM ELECTRONICS
Based on Lectures of Summer Schools

Stephen F. Jacobs, Marlan O. Scully, and Murray Sargent III, Editors

1973 Summer Schools

Vol. 1 **High Energy Lasers and Their Applications,** 1974
Edited by
Stephen F. Jacobs, Murray Sargent III, and Marlan O. Scully

Vol. 2 **Laser Applications to Optics and Spectroscopy,** in preparation
Edited by
Stephen F. Jacobs, Murray Sargent III, James F. Scott, and
Marlan O. Scully

Contributors

Petras V. Avizonis
Air Force Weapons Laboratory, Kirtland Air Force Base, New Mexico (pp. 247–292)

Keith Boyer
Los Alamos Scientific Laboratory, Los Alamos, New Mexico (pp. 293–332)

Paul W. Hoff
Lawrence Livermore Laboratories, University of California, Livermore, California (pp. 333–390)

Charles B. Hogge
Air Force Weapons Laboratory, Kirtland Air Force Base, New Mexico (pp. 177–246)

Frederic A. Hopf
Optical Sciences Center, University of Arizona, Tucson, Arizona (pp. 77–176)

Stephen F. Jacobs
Optical Sciences Center, University of Arizona, Tucson, Arizona (pp. 47–75)

Richard Morse
Los Alamos Scientific Laboratory, Los Alamos, New Mexico (pp. 391–406)

John R. Murray
Lawrence Livermore Laboratories, University of California, Livermore, California (pp. 333–390)

Murray Sargent III
Optical Sciences Center, University of Arizona, Tucson, Arizona (pp. 1–45)

Marlan O. Scully
Department of Physics and Optical Sciences Center, University of Arizona, Tucson, Arizona (pp. 47–75)

Hansen Shih
Optical Sciences Center, University of Arizona, Tucson, Arizona (pp. 47–75)

High Energy Lasers and Their Applications

Based on Lectures of the July 8–20, 1973 Summer School,
Crystal Mountain, Washington

Edited by
Stephen Jacobs, Murray Sargent III, and **Marlan O. Scully**
Optical Sciences Center, *University of Arizona, Tucson*

1974

Addison-Wesley Publishing Company
Advanced Book Program
Reading, Massachusetts

London · Amsterdam · Don Mills, Ontario · Sydney · Tokyo

Coden: **PHQEA**

Library of Congress Cataloging in Publication Data
Main entry under title:

High energy lasers and their applications.

(Physics of quantum electronics ; v. 1)
Summer school sponsored by the Optical Sciences
Center, University of Arizona.
  1. Lasers. I. Jacobs, Stephen, ed. II. Sargent,
Murray, ed. III. Scully, Marlan Orvil, 1939-   ed.
IV. Arizona. University. Optical Sciences Center.
V. Series.
TA1675.H53   621.36'6   74-26748
ISBN 0-201-05681-X

Reproduced by Addison-Wesley Publishing Company, Inc., Advanced Book Program, Reading,
Massachusetts, from camera-ready copy prepared by the office of the editors.

Copyright © 1974 by Addison-Wesley Publishing Company, Inc.
Published simultaneously in Canada.

Manufactured in the United States of America

For all high energy gas lasers temperature must
be controlled by flow rather than by conduction.
In this chapter we discuss three such lasers.

A review of the concept of controlled laser-
initiated fusion, including recent history of the
worldwide effort and an outline of the thermonuclear burn physics.

A brief overview of laser systems suitable for
concentrating large energies on a small thermonuclear target. Future excimer and quadrupole
transition lasers for fusion are discussed.

A long "back of the envelope" calculation to
convey orders of magnitude involved in laser
fusion.

This is the first volume of a new serial publication, Physics of Quantum Electronics. The contributions are based on lectures presented by well-known scientists at the Physics of Quantum Electronics Summer School. Sponsored by the Optical Sciences Center of The University of Arizona, this School is now held during alternate summers for two weeks in various scenic parts of the western United States. The current school is a tutorial symposium dealing with the frontiers in quantum electronics which has met at Flagstaff, Arizona (1968 and 1969) and at Prescott, Arizona (1971). The first two volumes are based on lectures given at Crystal Mountain, Washington, during the session of July 8-20, 1973.

The spirit of the school and of the publication is the presentation of recent developments in quantum electronics from first principles in order to enable workers specializing in one area to understand material in another. The contributors have been ever mindful of Peter Franken's admonition that generally such schools do not work because "physicists have a horror of saying anything that might appear to be too simple; for example, they say $P_1(\theta)$ instead of $\cos \theta$." The success of the summer school sessions indicates that the lecturers have avoided this pitfall. The regular lectures are given in the mornings and evenings. Afternoons are free for informal discussions in beautiful surroundings and for special seminars conducted by and for specialists in their fields of interest. In the past, the lecture notes had been published informally as Optical Science Center Technical Memoranda. The fact that these documents invariably disappeared with alacrity and that most articles found their ways into the various review journals led the editors to integrate the articles into volumes in this current endeavor.

This first volume concentrates on high energy lasers and their applications, notably on laser-induced fusion. The first chapter gives background theory for understanding laser operation with intense fields. The derivations are couched in intuitive terms, but nevertheless follow fairly rigorously from the underlying quantum mechanical foundations.

A number of new strong-signal formulas are presented, with graphs to illustrate tuning and pumping behavior. The second chapter deals with a very promising method of treating the unstable resonator, a device important for high energy laser operation due to the increased mode volume obtained. This method, too, is developed from first principles. Chapter 3 deals with amplifier theory in some detail, treating numerous amplifier configurations and media. After developing the theory in a fashion parallel to the laser treatment in Chapter 1, the author considers applications to molecular and solid-state lasers currently being used in fusion studies (discussed later in the volume). Chapter 4 deals with the propagation of intense laser beams in the atmosphere paying particular attention to problems of thermal blooming and atmospheric turbulence. Chapter 5 discusses the population inversion mechanisms in three important high power gas lasers: CO_2 electrical, CO_2 gas dynamic, and HF chemical.

The final three chapters of the book deal with laser-induced fusion. Chapter 6 gives a review of the basic concepts including an overview of the various international efforts to achieve this important phenomenon. Chapter 7 deals with the properties of lasers, both in principle and (present) practice that are relevant to inducing fusion. The final chapter presents a "back of the envelope" calculation that reveals the various orders of magnitude involved in laser fusion.

The editors are indebted to Kathleen Jacobs for her able handling of the school finances, to the typists, Kay Bergsten and Janet Rowe, for their tireless efforts, and to the many students whose comments and criticisms have improved the quality of the material significantly.

Stephen F. Jacobs
Murray Sargent III
Marlan O. Scully

Part A

LASER PHYSICS

STRONG SIGNAL LASER THEORY

Murray Sargent III

1.1. INTRODUCTION

In this chapter, we take a tour through strong-signal
laser theory from the foundations to the predictions. Our
trip will be something like a drive up a mountain with stops
along the way to examine the scenery. In this spirit, we
won't go into detailed derivations. They can be found, for
example, in the 1974 book *Laser Physics* by Marlan Scully,
Willis Lamb and myself.[1] Rather, we consider the important
equations, motivating them intuitively and illustrating them
numerically.

We wish to discuss two-mirror (henceforth standing
wave) and ring lasers as diagrammed in Fig. 1. Brewster
windows are indicated there to ensure that the laser field
is plane polarized, and therefore scalar in nature. We
describe laser operation with the semiclassical theory of
the interaction of radiation with matter. For this, the
electromagnetic field is treated classically according to a
set of Maxwell's equations that contain the polarization of
the laser medium induced by the field. This polarization is

1

derived from quantum mechanics. The method is depicted in
Fig. 2 explicitly illustrating the self-consistency requirement that the inducing field $\vec{E}'$ is, in fact, the same as the
sustained field $\vec{E}$.

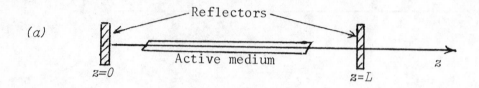

(a)

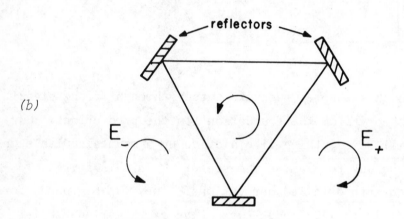

(b)

Fig. 1.   *(a) Diagram of laser showing reflectors in plane*
          perpendicular to laser (z) axis and active medium
          between reflectors. Brewster windows are sketched
          on the ends of the active medium to help enforce
          conditions that only one polarization component of
          the electric field exists as is assumed in this
          paper. (b) Corresponding ring laser configuration.
          Usually both running waves oscillate in a ring
          laser; unidirectional operation can be achieved by
          insertion of a device with high loss for one
          running wave in the cavity.

One subtlety in this procedure is the use of the
expectation value of an individual atomic dipole. Tradi-
tionally, this value is interpreted to yield the average

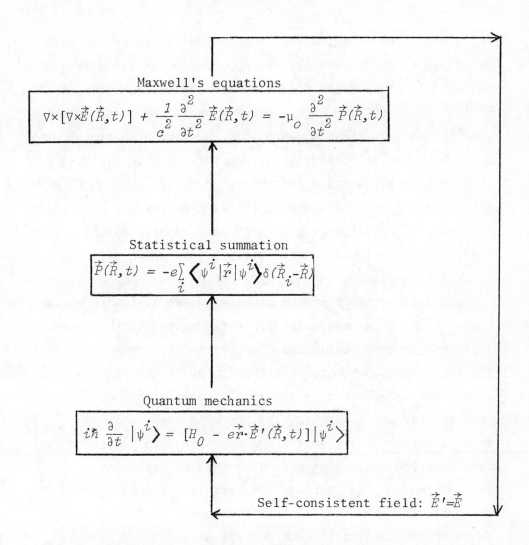

Fig. 2. *The semiclassical method. Self-consistent equations demonstrating that an assumed field $\vec{E}'(\vec{R},t)$ perturbs the ith atom according to the laws of quantum mechanics and induces an electric dipole expectation value. Values for atoms localized at $\vec{R}$ are added to yield macroscopic polarization, $\vec{P}(\vec{R},t)$. This polarization acts as a source in Maxwell's equations for a field $\vec{E}(\vec{R},t)$. The loop is completed by the self-consistency requirement that the field assumed, $\vec{E}'$, is equal to the field produced, $\vec{E}$.*

value from many measurements, a value which ordinarily differs from that of any single measurement. But since we are
adding up contributions from many closely spaced atoms, we
effectively obtain such an average anyhow. In fact, formally the semiclassical equations follow from a completely
quantum mechanical theory (i.e., field too) with the assumption of a coherent state for the field and neglect of some
tiny correlations. Suffice it to say that for our purposes,
the fully quantal theory gives the same results as the semiclassical, but with far more effort, so we again refer the
interested reader to Ref. 1.

   To further simplify our discussion, we 1) ignore variations in the electromagnetic field transverse to the laser
axis, and 2) suppose the field interacts with only two
levels of the quantum systems that comprise the laser's
active medium. We consider strong signal laser operation
both exactly and in the simpler, popular rate equation
approximation (REA). We further consider both homogeneously-
broadened and inhomogeneously-broadened active media.
Towards the end, we indicate what problems can be treated
with our techniques and what limitations seem to be inevi-
table in application to such devices as the gas dynamic
laser (GDL) and the transverse electronic, atmospheric (TEA)
lasers. The final portion of our tour consists of an overview of mode locking in quantum optics and is documented in
Ref. 2.

1.2. RELATION BETWEEN LASER FIELD AND POLARIZATION OF MEDIUM

   We suppose that the electromagnetic field in the laser
cavity can be represented by the scalar electric field

$E(z,t)$ written as the superposition of plane waves

$$E(z,t) = \frac{1}{2} \sum_n E_n(t) \exp[-i(\nu_n t + \phi_n)] U_n(z) + complex \atop conjugate.$$

(1)

Here the mode amplitudes $E_n(t)$ and phases $\phi_n(t)$ vary little in an optical frequency period and ν_n are the mode frequencies. The $U_n(z)$ specify the mode variations along the laser axis and consist of standing waves $[U_n(z) = \sin(K_n z)]$ for the two-mirror laser and running waves $[\exp(iK_n z)]$ for the ring laser. The wave number $K_n = n\pi/L$ or $2n\pi/L$ for the ring laser reflects the fact that there are an integral number of wavelengths in a round trip between mirrors. We take the polarization of the medium to be the corresponding superposition

$$P(z,t) = \frac{1}{2} \sum_n P_n(t) \exp[-i(\nu_n t + \phi_n)] U_n(z) + c.c.$$ (2)

in which the complex polarization component $P_n(t)$ also varies little in an optical frequency period. They are complex inasmuch as in general the induced polarization has different phase from the inducing field.

These quantities are then plugged into a suitable set of Maxwell's equations with careful attention to the slowly-varying properties of the E_n, ϕ_n and P_n, and with use of the orthogonality of the $U_n(z)$. The result is the "self-consistency" equations

$$\dot{E}_n \;=\; -\,\frac{1}{2}\,\frac{\nu_n}{Q_n}\,E_n \;-\; \frac{\nu_n}{2\varepsilon_o}\,\mathrm{Im}\{P_n\} \tag{3a}$$

$$\nu_n + \dot{\phi}_n \;=\; \Omega_n - \frac{\nu_n}{2\varepsilon_o}\,\mathrm{Re}\{P_n\}/E_n, \tag{3b}$$

so named because the field parameters ultimately appearing
in the formulas for the P_n are taken to be the very same as
the parameters in Eq. (1). The cavity Q's (determining mode
losses) are denoted by Q_n, and the passive cavity frequencies
$\Omega_n = c/K_n$.

It is worthwhile stopping at this point to gain a physical feel for these equations. The complex polarization P_n
is often related to the electric field component E_n by a
complex susceptibility χ_n, that is,

$$P_n \;=\; \varepsilon_o \chi_n E_n \;=\; \varepsilon_o (\chi_n{'} + i\chi_n{''})E_n. \tag{4}$$

For our problem, this susceptibility is itself a decreasing
function of the E_n inasmuch as the response of the laser
medium saturates. With (4), Eqs. (3) simplify to

$$\dot{E}_n \;=\; -\,\frac{1}{2}\,\frac{\nu_n}{Q_n}\,E_n \;-\; \frac{1}{2}\,\nu_n \chi_n{''} E_n \tag{5a}$$

$$\nu_n + \dot{\phi}_n \;=\; \Omega_n - \frac{1}{2}\,\nu_n \chi{'}. \tag{5b}$$

Equation (5a) expresses energy conservation (and could
plausibly be postulated therefrom). To see this, note that
the mode energy h_n is proportional to $E_n{}^2$. Hence multiplication of (5a) by $2E_n$ yields the energy time rate of change

$$\dot{h}_n \;=\; -\,\frac{\nu_n}{Q_n}\,h_n \;-\; \nu_n \chi_n{}'' h_n$$

$$=\; -\,\underbrace{\frac{\text{cavity losses}}{\text{second}}} \;+\; \underbrace{\frac{\text{medium gain}}{\text{second}}} \;(\chi_n{}'' < 0).$$

In particular for single mode operation, the gain parameter $\chi_n{}''$ saturates sufficiently in time to yield an energy gain/second equal in magnitude to the cavity losses/second. At this point steady-state laser operation is achieved.

Inasmuch as the susceptibility term $\chi_n{}'$ is small compared to unity, the frequency-determining equation (5b) can be "summed" to give

$$\nu_n + \dot{\phi}_n \;=\; \frac{\Omega_n}{1 + \chi_n{}'/2} \;=\; \frac{\Omega_n}{\eta}\,,$$

where η is the index of refraction. This equation [or (5b)] reveals a curious difference between the gain problem and the classical absorption problem, namely that the oscillation *frequency* is shifted by the medium instead of the *wavelength*. This results from the self-consistent nature of the laser field which requires an integral number of wavelengths in a round trip regardless of the medium characteristics.

Linear values of $\chi_n{}'$ and $\chi_n{}''$ are graphed in Fig. 3 for a homogeneously broadened medium having the line center $\omega[\neq 2\pi\nu!]$. Note that both curves are negative with respect to the classical absorption curves. In addition to gain, this change of sign leads to mode pulling: ν_n is closer to ω than is the passive frequency Ω_n in contrast to the dispersive nature one expects of absorbers.

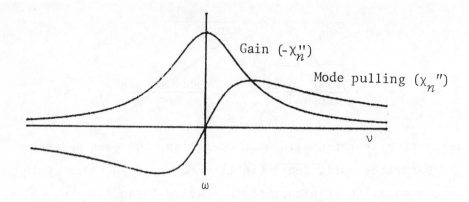

*Fig. 3. Gain and mode pulling parts of the complex
          susceptibility of (4) for a homogeneously
          broadened medium (Lorentzian gain).*

1-3. EQUATIONS OF MOTION FOR LASER MEDIUM

The next leg of our journey concerns the response of
the active atoms (or molecules) to the laser electric field.
The two relevant levels of the medium we consider are
depicted in Fig. 4. There N_a is the number of atoms in the
upper level, N_b, the number in the lower level, λ_a is the
rate (no/sec assumed to be constant) at which atoms are
pumped to the upper level (λ_b to the lower), and $\gamma_a N_a$ is the
rate of decay from the upper level due to spontaneous emis-
sion and collisions. The transfer between levels due to the
interaction with the laser field is represented there in the
rate equation approximation (REA) discussed in Sec. 4. The
transfer rate is given by the rate constant R multiplied by
the population difference $N_a - N_b$.

The time development of the atomic response is written
most easily with some additional notation. Specifically, we
define the interaction energy

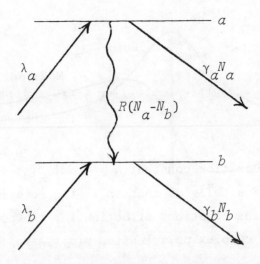

Fig. 4. *Energy level diagram for two-level atoms comprising laser's active medium. The resonance frequency for the transition is ω. Diagram depicts flow given by rate equations (18).*

$$V_{ab} = -\frac{1}{2} \wp \sum_n E_n(t) \exp[-i(\nu_n t + \phi_n)] U_n(z) \qquad (6)$$

and write the polarization (2) in the form

$$P(z,t) = \frac{1}{2} p(z,t) + \text{c.c.}, \qquad (7)$$

where $p(z,t)$ is the positive frequency part (that going like $e^{-\nu t}$), and $\wp$, pronounced "squiggle," is the electric-dipole matrix element.[†] The complex polarization component $P_n(t)$

_____

[†]The complex polarization $p(z,t)$ is $\wp \rho_{ab}(z,t)$, where $\rho_{ab}(z,t)$ is an unnormalized density matrix element. Similarly N_a is ρ_{aa}. See the appendix for a derivation of Eqs. (4) from quantum mechanics.

of (2) is then given by

$$P_n(t) = 2 \exp[i(\nu_n t + \phi_n)] \frac{1}{N} \int_0^L dz U_n^*(z) p(z,t) \qquad (8)$$

with the normalization constant $N = \int_0^L dz |U_n(z)|^2$. Then quantum mechanics tells us that in the rotating wave approximation the equations of motion for the populations N_a and N_b and the complex polarization $p(z,t)$ are

$$\dot{p} = -(i\omega + \gamma)p + \frac{i}{\hbar} V_{ab}[N_a - N_b]\wp \qquad (9a)$$

$$\dot{N}_a = \lambda_a - \gamma_a N_a - [\frac{i}{\hbar} V_{ab} p^* + \text{c.c.}]/\wp \qquad (9b)$$

$$\dot{N}_b = \lambda_b - \gamma_b N_b + [\frac{i}{\hbar} V_{ab} p^* + \text{c.c.}]/\wp . \qquad (9c)$$

Here γ is the decay constant for the polarization p and is ordinarily larger than the average of γ_a and γ_b, since there are collisions which cause the induced dipole moment to de-phase, i.e., decay, without change in the probabilities of level occupancy. The γ_α and $\gamma_\alpha N_\alpha$ ($\alpha = a,b$) terms in (9) are plausible in view of the flow diagram in Fig. 4, but how can we understand the terms due to the atom-field interaction? From (9b) and (9c) we see, at least, that what leaves the upper level due to this stimulated emission ends up in the lower level (terms are equal in magnitude and opposite in sign), but it's not clear in this form just how the field drives the atoms. We consider this question first from a pictorial point of view obtaining what are known as

"Bloch-like" equations. This development is helpful also
for the pulse propagation discussion of Fred Hopf given
in Chap. 3.   We consider second (in Sec. 4) a
different limit (large γ) known as the rate equation approximation.

Suppose first for simplicity that the field is a
single-mode field, so that

$$V_{ab} = -\frac{\wp}{2} E_n \exp[-i(\nu_n t + \phi_n)] U_n(z)$$

and $p(z,t) = P(z,t)\exp[-i(\nu_n t + \phi_n)]$. Then the equations of
motion (9) reduce to

$$\dot{P} = -(i\omega - i\nu_n + \gamma)P - \frac{i}{2\hbar}\wp^2 E_n[N_a - N_b] \tag{10a}$$

$$\dot{N}_a = \lambda_a - \gamma_a N_a - [\frac{i}{2\hbar} E_n P^* + \text{c.c.}] \tag{10b}$$

and a similar equation for $\dot{N}_b$. We further choose equal
level decay times, $\gamma_b = \gamma_a = 1/T_1$ and use the traditional
Bloch time T_2 for $1/\gamma$. Finally we define the slowly-varying
components of the three-dimensional vector $\vec{R}$ by

$$R_1 - iR_2 = P_n/\wp N \tag{11a}$$

$$R_3 = (N_a - N_b)/N, \tag{11b}$$

where N is the number of atoms. With these substitutions
and neglect of the pump, the equations of motion (9)

become the "Bloch-like" versions

$$\dot{R}_1 = -(\omega - \nu_n)R_2 - R_1/T_2 \tag{12a}$$

$$\dot{R}_2 = (\omega - \nu_n)R_1 - R_2/T_2 + \wp E_n R_3/\hbar \tag{12b}$$

$$\dot{R}_3 = -\wp E_n R_2/\hbar - R_3/T_1. \tag{12c}$$

To see what $\vec{R}$ is doing, suppose $T_2 = T_1$. Then (12) can be written as the vector equation

$$\dot{\vec{R}} = \vec{R} \times \vec{B} - \vec{R}/T_1, \tag{13}$$

where the "effective field" is given by

$$\vec{B} = (\wp E_n/\hbar)\hat{e}_1 - (\omega - \nu_n)\hat{e}_3. \tag{14}$$

Now we have a picture (Fig. 5), for Eq. (13) describes the rotation of $\vec{R}$ about $\vec{B}$ as it decays away due to the T_1 processes. In particular for resonance ($\nu_n = \omega$), zero decay ($T_1 = \infty$) and for an initial $R_3(0) = 1$ (all atoms in upper state), $\vec{R}$ rotates down to $-\hat{e}_3$ and back up under the influence of the "field" $\wp E_n/\hbar$. In Bloch's problem of nuclear magnetic resonance (NMR), the picture has an immediate significance, for $\vec{R}$ times the magnetic dipole moment is, in fact, just the magnetization of the medium involved and its rotation is in the space we live in. The electric-dipole case is not so tangible, but the analogy holds and one can visualize the electric field forcing the atom to flop back and forth between the levels in a coherent fashion.

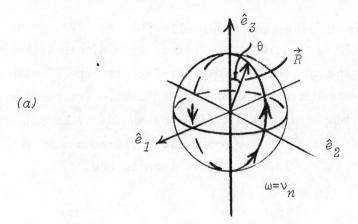

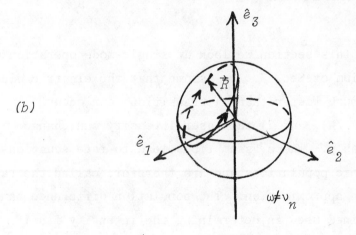

Fig. 5.   (a) For central tuning $(\omega - \nu_n)$ and $\wp < 0$ (for elec-
          tron), $\vec{R}$ precesses clockwise about $\hat{e}_1$ at angular
          frequency $\wp E_n / \hbar$ as determined by Eq. (13). The
          electric-dipole interaction energy is directed
          along the $\hat{e}_1$ axis in the rotating wave approxima-
          tion. For an initial $R_3(0) = -1$ (system in lower
          level), $R_3(\pi \hbar / \wp E_n) = 1$, that is, the atom makes a
          transition in a time $\pi \hbar / \wp E_n$. For some detuning
          $(\omega \neq \nu_n)$, $\vec{R}$ acquires a nonzero $\hat{e}_1$ component and a
          complete transition never occurs (e.g., from upper
          to lower level). $\vec{R}$ precesses clockwise about the
          effective "field" $\vec{B}$ of (14) with frequency $|\vec{B}| =$
          $[(\omega - \nu_n)^2 + (\wp E_n / \hbar)^2]^{\frac{1}{2}}$, thus tracing out a cone in
          the rotating frame.

Although it isn't explicitly apparent from (9), we see from
our little derivation that the electric-dipole interaction
term in the complex, rapidly-varying versions (9) also
attempts to drive the atoms up and down. Its success is, of
course, tempered by the excitation and decay terms, even to
the point where the net population difference can remain
constant. This is the case we turn to now.

1.4.   SINGLE-MODE OPERATION IN THE RATE EQUATION

       APPROXIMATION (REA)

In this section we look at single-mode operation with
the medium of Sec. 3. We assume that the electric dipole
decays much faster than 1) transitions can occur
$(\gamma \gg \wp E_n/\hbar)$, and 2) the laser intensity can change
appreciably. These assumptions lead to rate equations for
the atomic populations and are therefore called the rate
equation approximation. The population difference can then
be obtained used in determining the intensity itself. This
approach is the simplest case of strong signal laser theory
(even of laser theory in general) and provides a reference
for all other theories.

First we note that by multiplying Eq. (9a) by the integrating factor $\exp[(i\omega+\gamma)t]$, the resulting equation can be
solved formally for the complex polarization p as

$$p(z,t) = i\frac{\wp}{\hbar}\int_{-\infty}^{t} dt'\, V_{ab}(z,t') \tag{15}$$

$$\times \exp[-(i\omega+\gamma)(t-t')][N_a(z,t') - N_b(z,t')].$$

For single mode in (1), with (6) for V_{ab} and the assumptions that the amplitude E_n, phase ϕ_n and population difference $N_a - N_b$ vary little in the time $1/\gamma$, the polarization becomes

$$p(z,t) \quad = \quad -i \frac{\wp^2}{2\hbar} E_n \exp[-i(\nu_n t + \phi_n)] U_n(z) [N_a - N_b] \mathcal{D}(\omega - \nu_n),$$

$$\tag{16}$$

in which $\mathcal{D}(\Delta)$ is a convenient abbreviation for a frequently occurring denominator

$$\mathcal{D}_x(\Delta) \quad = \quad \frac{1}{\gamma_x + i\Delta} \, , \quad x \ = \ a, \ b \text{ or missing.} \tag{17}$$

We now plug this formula for $p(z,t)$ into the equations of motion (9b) and (9c) for the populations and find the rate equations[†]

$$\dot{N}_a \quad = \quad \lambda_a - \gamma_a N_a - R[N_a - N_b] \tag{18a}$$

$$\dot{N}_b \quad = \quad \lambda_b - \gamma_b N_b + R[N_a - N_b], \tag{18b}$$

where the rate constant $R(z)$ is given by

$$R(z) \quad = \quad \frac{1}{2} (\wp E_n / \hbar)^2 |U_n(z)|^2 \frac{1}{\gamma} L(\omega - \nu_n), \tag{19}$$

[†]These rate equations are generalizations of the well-known Einstein (A & B) discussion used, for example, by Dienes in Chap. 2 of Vol. 2.

and the dimensionless Lorentzian

$$L_x(\Delta) = \frac{\gamma_x^2}{\gamma_x^2 + \Delta^2} . \tag{20}$$

These rate equations correspond to the flows depicted in Fig. 4.

In steady-state operation ($\dot{N}_a = \dot{N}_b = 0$), Eqs. (18) can be solved for the population difference:

$$N_a - N_b = \frac{N(z,t)}{1 + 2(\gamma_{ab}/\gamma)I_n |U_n(z)|^2 L(\omega-\nu_n)} . \tag{21}$$

Here we have introduced the very useful dimensionless intensity

$$I_n = \frac{1}{2}(\wp E_n/\hbar)^2 (\gamma_a \gamma_b)^{-1}, \tag{22}$$

which buries an often unknown constant ($\wp$) and leads to uniformity in the various laser treatments. The $N(z,t)$ is the unsaturated ($R = I_n = 0$) population difference

$$N(z,t) = \frac{\gamma_a}{\gamma_a} - \frac{\gamma_b}{\gamma_b} . \tag{23}$$

In this steady-state situation, the appropriate $\vec{R}$ vector (Sec. 3) assumes a constant position in the $\hat{e}_1$, $\hat{e}_2$, $\hat{e}_3$ space, rather than rotating around. The position depends on the competing effects of excitation, decay and induced transitions.

The saturated difference (21) contains a $|U_n(z)|^2$ modulation in the saturation factor. For the unidirectional ring laser, this factor is unity and that laser is often treated in the textbooks because of its consequent simplicity. For the standing wave case, the factor is $\sin^2 K_n z$, which leads to "spatial holes" burned in the population difference by the peaks of the standing-wave intensity (Fig. 6). We meet this hole burning concept in a velocity context in the gas laser discussion of Sec. 5.[3] The amount of saturation for a given intensity is proportional to $(\gamma_{ab}/\gamma\gamma_a\gamma_b)$. Inasmuch as the γ's increase as pressure (especially γ itself), higher pressures yield smaller saturation. This, in turn, leads to a larger steady-state intensity [see Eq. (38)].

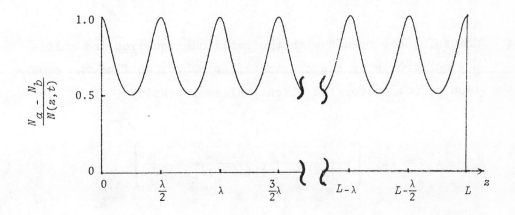

Fig. 6. *Normalized population difference versus axial co-*
ordinate. Spatial holes burned by the laser field
in this difference are clearly depicted. Eq. (21)
was used with $|U_n(z)|^2 = \sin^2 K_n z$. For $2\gamma_{ab} = \gamma$ and
central tuning $(\omega = \nu_n)$, this figure corresponds to
$I_n = 1$, which is not an uncommon value in lasers.

The population difference (21) can be combined with the complex polarization (16) and with (8) for the polarization component $P_n(t)$ giving

$$P_n(t) = -i\frac{\wp^2}{\hbar}E_n D(\omega-\nu_n)\frac{1}{N}\int_0^L dz\left[\frac{N(z,t)|U_n(z)|^2}{1+2(\gamma_{ab}/\gamma)I_n L(\omega-\nu_n)|U_n(z)|}\right]$$

(24)

Let's consider operation for two cases, the unidirectional ring and standing-wave lasers. For the former, $|U_n(z)|^2 = 1$, and (24) can be written simply in terms of the average unsaturated population difference

$$\overline{N} = \frac{1}{L}\int_0^L dz N(z,t)|U_n(z)|^2.$$

(25)

Combining the result with the amplitude equation and multiplying through by the constant $(\hbar/\wp)^2\gamma_a\gamma_b$, we find the equation of motion for the dimensionless intensity

$$\dot{I}_n = 2I_n\left[\frac{g}{1 + 2(\gamma_{ab}/\gamma)L(\omega-\nu_n)I_n} - \frac{\nu_n}{2Q_n}\right]$$

(26)

where the linear gain parameter

$$g = (\nu^2\overline{N}/2\varepsilon_o\hbar\gamma)L(\omega-\nu_n).$$

(27)

This gain parameter is most conveniently written in terms of the relative excitation (excitation relative to threshold excitation)

$$\mathcal{N} = \overline{N}/\overline{N}_T,$$ (28)

as

$$g = \frac{\nu_n}{2Q_n} \mathcal{N}L(\omega-\nu_n).$$ (29)

In (26) we see quite simply the effect of saturation. For small intensity, there is exponential buildup with the factor $\exp[2(g - \frac{1}{2}\nu_n/Q_n)t]$. As I_n builds up, the gain term is reduced by the increasing denominator, representing the fact that the atoms only have a finite amount of energy to offer. Eventually a steady-state ($\dot{I}_n = 0$) is reached when the saturated gain equals the cavity losses. The intensity for this case is

$$I_n = \frac{\mathcal{N}L(\omega-\nu_n) - 1}{2(\gamma_{ab}/\gamma)L(\omega-\nu_n)}.$$ (30)

This is illustrated in Fig. 7 for a number of relative excitation values.

The solution for the standing-wave laser is not as simple due to the presence of the $\sin^2 K_n z$ factor in the denominator of the integrand of (24) for $p(z,t)$. The integral was evaluated by Lamb,[4] and with some careful algebra, one can show (new result) that the steady-state intensity is given by

$$I_n = \frac{\mathscr{N}L(\omega-\nu_n) - \frac{1}{4} - \frac{1}{4}\sqrt{8\mathscr{N}L(\omega-\nu_n)+1}}{(\gamma_{ab}/\gamma)L(\omega-\nu_n)} \qquad (31)$$

This expression is admittedly not as transparent as (30), although it is quite amenable to computer evaluation.

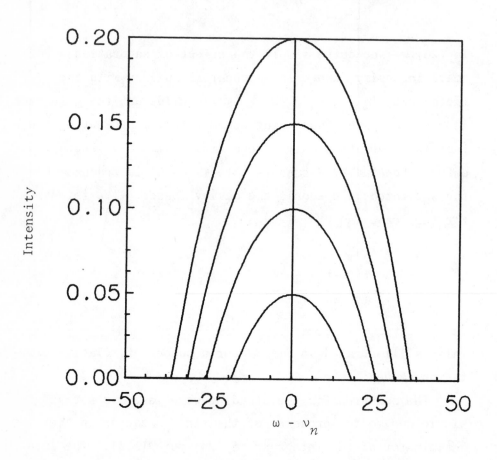

Fig. 7.   *Graphs of single-mode (dimensionless) intensity (30) versus detuning* $(\omega-\nu_n)$ *for homogeneously broadened* $(\gamma=2\pi\times100\mathrm{MHz},\ \gamma_{ab}=2\pi\times50\mathrm{MHz}),$ *stationary atoms. The relative excitation* $\mathscr{N}$ *of Eq. (28) are (in order of increasing maxima) 1.05, 1.10, 1.15, and 1.2.*

1-5.   LASER OPERATION WITH INHOMOGENEOUSLY BROADENED MEDIA

Many laser media are inhomogeneously broadened, that is, different atoms have different line centers as suggested in Fig. 8. This kind of broadening differs from the homogeneous

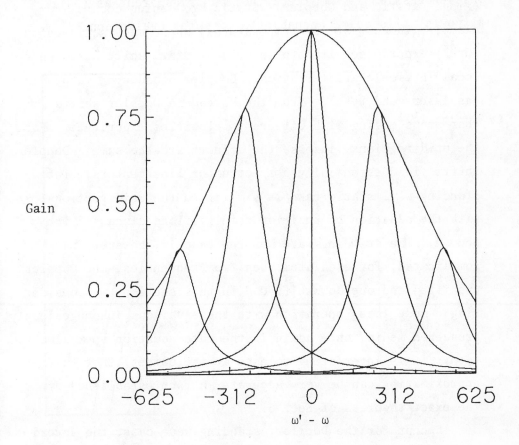

Fig. 8.   Graph showing individual atomic response curves superimposed on inhomogeneously broadened line for possible laser medium. The homogeneous contribution to the medium linewidth is 150 MHz; the inhomogeneous contribution, 1000 MHz. As such, the medium is primarily inhomogeneously broadened.

variety considered in preceding sections in that it is a
dynamical (not random) property and can be reversed. A
famous example of this is photon echo (which, by the way,
can be explained without reference to photons). We consider
here two basically different kinds of inhomogeneous broadening: static and Doppler. Static broadening occurs, for
example, in ruby at low temperatures, where each active atom
(Cr^{3+}) experiences its own individual Stark shift based on
local lattice characteristics. Doppler broadening occurs in
gas lasers and results from the spread in Doppler shifts
that atoms moving with different velocities experience. For
the unidirectional lasers, the effects are the same: Doppler
shifts yield essentially a spectrum of line centers. The
standing-wave static case is similar to the unidirectional
with the addition of position complications discussed in
Sec. 4. The standing-wave *Doppler* case is, however, more
complicated, for each atom sees two frequencies, one Doppler
upshifted and one downshifted. In this section, we consider
single-mode laser operation with these various inhomogeneously
broadened media, once again in the rate equation approximation. It is interesting to note at the outset, that this
approximation can be very accurate, a fact established by
the exact theories of Sec. 6.

Except for the Doppler, standing-wave case, the spread
of line centers in the inhomogeneously broadened medium is
represented in the theory by a line-center dependence in the
level populations, $N_a(z,\omega',t)$ and $N_b(z,\omega',t)$ and in the complex polarization $p(z,\omega',t)$. The equations of motion are
still given by (9). The macroscopic polarization $P(z,t)$,
however, is contributed to by all systems at z at time t regardless of ω' and hence includes an integral over the
latter:

$$P(z,t) = \frac{1}{2} \int d\omega' p(z,\omega',t) + \text{c.c.} \tag{32}$$

Furthermore, the linear population inversion includes a function specifying the nature of the inhomogeneity, namely

$$N(z,\omega',t) = W(\omega')N(z,t). \tag{33}$$

For many media, the Maxwellian distribution

$$W(\omega') = \frac{1}{\Delta\omega\sqrt{\pi}} \exp[-(\omega'-\omega)^2/(\Delta\omega)^2] \tag{34}$$

is descriptive and we use it in most situations. With these additions, we can take over the homogeneously broadened results of Sec. 4 immediately. Combining Eqs. (32), (24) and (8), we find the complex polarization component

$$P_n(t) = -i \frac{\wp^2}{\hbar} E_n \frac{1}{N} \int_0^L dz N(z,t) |U_n(z)|^2$$

$$\times \int_{-\infty}^{\infty} d\omega' \frac{W(\omega')\mathcal{D}(\omega'-\nu_n)}{1+2(\gamma_{ab}/\gamma)I_n L(\omega'-\nu_n)|U_n(z)|^2} . \tag{35}$$

For the unidirectional cases, $|U_n(z)|^2 = 1$ as usual, leading to $\bar{N}$ for the z integration. The frequency integral is conveniently expressed in terms of the plasma dispersion function defined by

$$Z(\gamma+i\omega-i\nu_n) = \frac{i}{\sqrt{\pi}} \int_{-\infty}^{\infty} d\omega' \; \exp[-(\omega'-\omega)^2/(\Delta\omega)^2] \mathcal{D}(\omega'-\nu_n).$$

$$(36)$$

Specifically, we find by the method of partial fractions (and some manipulations)

$$P_n(t) = -\frac{\wp^2}{\hbar\Delta\omega} \bar{N} E_n [Z_r(\gamma'+i\omega-i\nu_n)$$

$$+ i \frac{\gamma}{\gamma'} Z_i(\gamma'+i\omega-i\nu_n)], \qquad (37)$$

where the *power* broadened decay constant

$$\gamma' = \gamma\sqrt{1 + 2(\gamma_{ab}/\gamma)I_n} \qquad (38)$$

and Z_r and Z_i are the real and imaginary parts of Z.

These parts resemble the Lorentzian versions of Fig. 3, but with a Gaussian influence (more so as $\gamma/\Delta\omega \to 0$) near line center. The presence of the power broadened γ' in (37) reduces the magnitudes of both parts below the corresponding γ value, that is, the polarization saturates. In addition, the imaginary term (giving the gain) contains the additional saturation factor γ/γ'. The intensity equation of motion is given from (3a) and (37) by

$$\dot{I}_n = 2I_n \frac{\nu_n}{2Q_n} \left[\frac{\gamma}{\gamma'} \mathcal{N} \frac{Z_i(\gamma'+i\omega-i\nu_n)}{Z_i(\gamma)} - 1 \right]. \qquad (39)$$

Here we see that the steady-state condition $\dot{I}_n = 0$ yields a transcendental equation in I_n and must be solved in general numerically. This is characteristic of strong-signal theories involving inhomogeneously broadened media. We note, however, that in the homogeneously broadened limit, Eq. (39) reduces to the earlier Eq. (26), and that the extreme inhomogeneity limit ($\Delta\omega \gg \gamma'$) approximates $Z_i(\gamma + i\Delta)$ by $\sqrt{\pi} \exp[-\Delta^2/(\Delta\omega)^2]$. The steady-state condition for (39) then can be solved as

$$I_n = 2\,\frac{\gamma}{\gamma_{ab}}\,\left[\mathcal{N}^2 \exp[-2(\omega - \nu_n)^2/(\Delta\omega)^2] - 1 \right]. \tag{40}$$

This shows a truncated Gaussian dependence on detuning in contrast to the truncated Lorentzian dependence of the homogeneous case in Fig. 7.

For the static broadened, standing-wave case, the frequency integral can be performed independently of the z integration, but the I_n in (38) is multiplied by $\sin^2 K_n z$. I do not know how to do the resulting z integration over the plasma dispersion function, so I leave it as an exercise for the student. It is, of course, possible to solve for the intensity to third order in the electric-dipole interaction energy, but this is a set of lectures on strong-signal theory.

We come now to the more complicated standing-wave, Doppler broadened case. The irony is that I can do the final integral for this allegedly harder case! For this problem, we use the axial component v of velocity in place of ω' for the inhomogeneity variable and write the frequency distribution $W(\omega')$ in terms of v as

$$W(v) = \frac{1}{u\sqrt{\pi}} \exp(-v^2/u^2),$$

where u is the most probable speed of the gas atoms (or molecules). The width parameter $\Delta\omega$ is replaced by the frequency Ku. The equations of motion are again given by (9) in which the time derivative (dot) stands for the convective derivative $(\partial/\partial t) + v(\partial/\partial z)$.

First note that the standing wave is the sum of two oppositely directed running waves:

$$E_n \cos\nu_n t \, \sin K_n z = \frac{1}{2} E_n \, [\sin(\nu_n t + K_n z)$$

$$- \sin(\nu_n t - K_n z)].$$

Hence an atom subject to this field moving with an axial component v sees *two* frequencies given by $\nu_n(1 \pm v/c)$ as indicated in Fig. 9a. Formally this creates two holes burned in the population difference, now versus v (Fig. 9b); the rate constant R of (19) is replaced by the value

$$R(v) = \frac{1}{8} (\wp E_n/\hbar)^2 \frac{1}{\gamma} [L(\omega-\nu_n+Kv) + L(\omega-\nu_n-Kv)]. \qquad (41)$$

The rate equations for the populations $N_a(z,v,t)$ and $N_b(z,v,t)$ have the same form as the stationary case (18). In (41), we have replaced the $|U_n(z)|^2 = \sin^2 K_n z$ factor by the average value 1/2 that a rapidly moving atom would experience. This approximation is not as good near line center

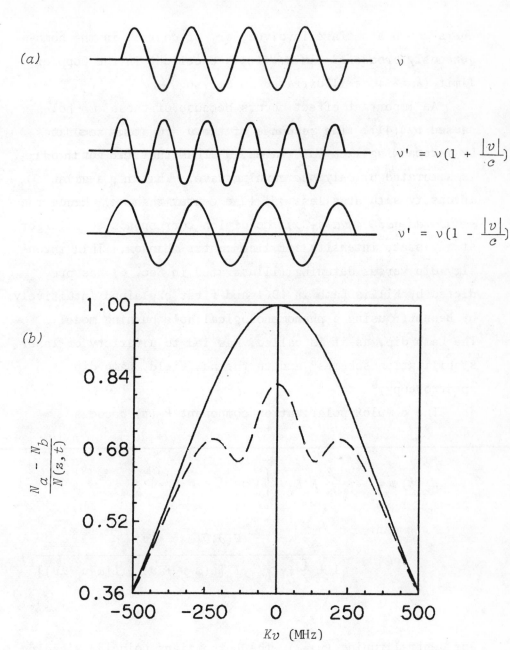

Fig. 9.   (a) Drawing showing how traveling wave with oscil-
          lation frequency ν appears Doppler downshifted to
          an atom moving the same direction as wave and up-
          shifted to atom moving other way. (b) Unsaturated
          (solid) and saturated (dahsed) population differ-
          ence $N_a - N_b$ vs. z component of velocity.   Formula
          used is $\{1 + R(v) 2\gamma_{ab}/\gamma_a \gamma_b\}^{-\frac{1}{2}}$. Drawing depicts holes
          burned by field intensity for $v = \pm c(1 - \omega/\nu)$.

where $v \simeq 0$ atoms are involved, or, of course, in the homogeneously broadened limit. It is excellent in the Doppler limit $(Ku >> \gamma)$ as illustrated in Sec. 6.

An important effect occurs because of these *two* holes caused by (41). The response of the $v \simeq 0$ atoms saturates by interacting with *both* waves, whereas that for nonzero v is saturated by only *one* running wave. That is, a given intensity saturates less *off* line center than *on*. Hence the *saturated-gain-equals-loss* condition corresponds to a larger steady-state intensity off line center than on. This intensity dip versus detuning (illustrated in Sec. 6) was predicted by Willis Lamb in 1961 and first explained intuitively by Bennett[3] using a phenomenological hole burning model. The Lamb dip, as it is called, has led to a variety of laser stabilization schemes[5] and to the new field, Lamb dip spectroscopy.[6]

The complex polarization component $P_n(t)$ becomes

$$P_n(t) = -i \, \frac{\wp^2}{\hbar} \, \bar{N} \, E_n \int_{-\infty}^{\infty} dv$$

$$\times \frac{W(v) \mathcal{D}(\omega - \nu_n + Kv)}{1 + \frac{1}{2} (\gamma_{ab}/\gamma) I_n [L(\omega - \nu_n + Kv) + L(\omega - \nu_n - Kv)]} \, .$$

$$(42)$$

For central tuning $(\nu_n = \omega)$, the Lorentzians coincide yielding an integral just like that for the unidirectional case (35) for central tuning, but without the factor of 2 in the denominator. Hence the intensity equation of motion is just (39) with $\nu_n = \omega$ and the power broadened γ' replaced by the value $\gamma \sqrt{1 + (\gamma_{ab}/\gamma) I_n}$. Off line center, the algebra is

considerably trickier. We give here only the result and
refer the interested reader to Prob. 8-12 of Ref. 1 for the
method. We find ($\Delta \equiv \omega - \nu_n$)

$$P_n(t) = -\frac{\wp^2}{\hbar Ku} \bar{N} E_n \frac{\gamma + i\Delta}{2} \left\{ [1 + A] \left[\frac{Z(\upsilon_+)}{\upsilon_+} \right] \right.$$

$$\left. + [1 - A] \left[\frac{Z(\upsilon_-)}{\upsilon_-} \right] \right\}, \quad (43)$$

where the complex frequencies

$$\upsilon_\pm^2 = \gamma'^2 - \Delta^2 \pm \frac{1}{2} \sqrt{(\gamma\gamma_{ab}I_n)^2 - 16\Delta^2\gamma'^2} ,$$

the factor

$$A = \frac{\gamma_{ab}I_n + i\Delta}{\sqrt{(\gamma_{ab}I_n)^2 - 16\Delta^2\gamma'^2/\gamma^2}}$$

and the power broadened γ

$$\gamma' = \gamma\sqrt{1 + \frac{1}{2}(\gamma_{ab}/\gamma)I_n}.$$

Unfortunately it isn't easy to separate real and imaginary
parts of (43) for use in the self-consistency equations (3),
even in the Doppler limit. But (44) is quite amenable to
numerical analysis. Note that here we obtain a

transcendental equation for I_n most inexorably, since I_n is buried in γ' all over the place. This requires the use of a Newton-Raphson iterative method (or equivalent) for computations of the steady-state intensity.

1.6. "EXACT" STRONG SIGNAL LASER THEORIES

The exact theories still involve, of course, some basic approximations such as the rotating wave and semiclassical approximations. But they remove assumptions such as rapid atomic decay in times for which the electric field or population difference can change appreciably (REA). The methods proceed on the basis of Fourier analysis as delineated towards the end of this section. We are principally interested in the single-mode, standing-wave Doppler-broadened laser,[7,8,9,10] the two-mode bidirectional ring laser,[11] and the two-mode unidirectional ring laser. Our approach treats all three in a uniform fashion even allowing extensions to the multimode, modelocked cases. Inasmuch as the algebra is fierce, I present the material on an intuitive level and refer the reader to a forthcoming publication[12] for the details.

Consider first the standing-wave Doppler laser of Sec. 5. Atoms moving with nonzero v see two frequencies. Inasmuch as a nonlinear medium is involved, the population difference $D(z,v,t) \equiv N_a(z,v,t) - N_b(z,v,t)$ develops pulsations at multiples of $2Kv$. These pulsations act like "Raman" shifters coupling and generating polarization components induced at the array of frequencies depicted in Fig. 10. We do not see these pulsations in the laser output, of course, since v is integrated over, but their presence changes the intensity

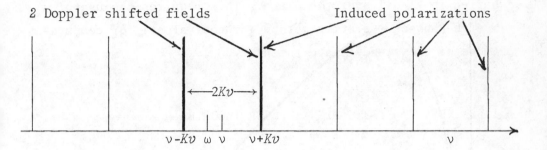

2 Doppler shifted fields   Induced polarizations

$\leftarrow 2Kv \rightarrow$

$v-Kv\ \ \omega\ v\ \ \ \ v+Kv$ v

Fig. 10.   Diagram of polarization components generated in
nonlinear Doppler broadened medium by single-mode
standing wave field.

from the REA analysis of Sec. 5 particularly for small v
situations (near and at central tuning). They are also neglected in Bennett's hole burning analysis,[3] which is something like the REA method, although more phenomenological.
In particular, the single hole burned by the two running
waves for central tuning exhibits a bump in its middle as
illustrated in Fig. 11.   Intuitively we can understand the
reduced saturation indicated by the bump by noting that zero
v atoms are involved for which spatial holes (Fig. 6) are
important. These holes are assumed to wash out in the REA
analysis [see Eq. (41)] and lead to a reduced average (over
z) saturation, that is, a bump. The degree to which the
spatial holes actually do wash out is illustrated in Fig. 12.

The hole in population difference versus v is not the
Lamb dip, of course, which occurs in the intensity versus
detuning curves. The latter is illustrated in Fig. 13 for a
number of relative excitations.   In Fig. 14, the REA results
are compared to the exact revealing considerably more deviation for central tuning than elsewhere, although the

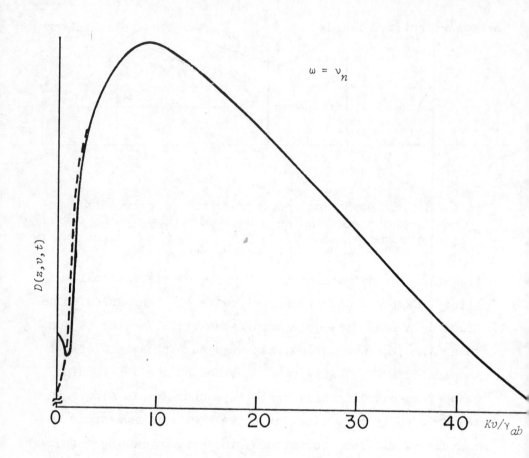

$$\omega = \nu_n$$

$D(z,v,t)$

Kv/γ_{ab}

Fig. 11. Population difference versus axial component v of velocity in exact and REA treatments. The former features the bump in the bottom of the hole burned by the standing-wave field. From Stenholm and Lamb.[8]

agreement is really quite good for both considering the huge values of relative excitation involved.

The bidirectional ring laser is very similar to the standing-wave Doppler device, but the amplitudes of the two running waves are no longer constrained to be equal, nor is a static phase relationship required. In fact, a cavity

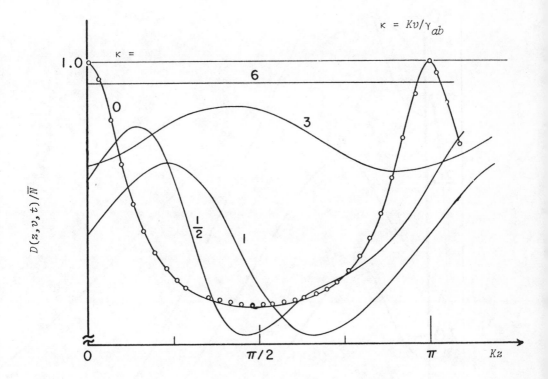

Fig. 12.   *Normalized population difference versus spatial pahse Kz along laser axis. Spatial holes burned by field intensity for nonmoving atoms are seen to wash out for rapidly moving atoms. In this and the following two figures, large Doppler inhomogeneity is used (Ku>>γ) and γ = γ_ab. From Stenholm and Lamb.* [8]

rotation can change the frequencies substantially and provide a practical scheme for a gyroscope. The nonlinear beating occurs between two frequencies seen by an atom, this time with value $\nu_- - \nu_+ + 2Kv$. The array of generated polarization components is depicted in Fig. 15a. Numerical calculations have been completed on this case as reported in Ref. 12.

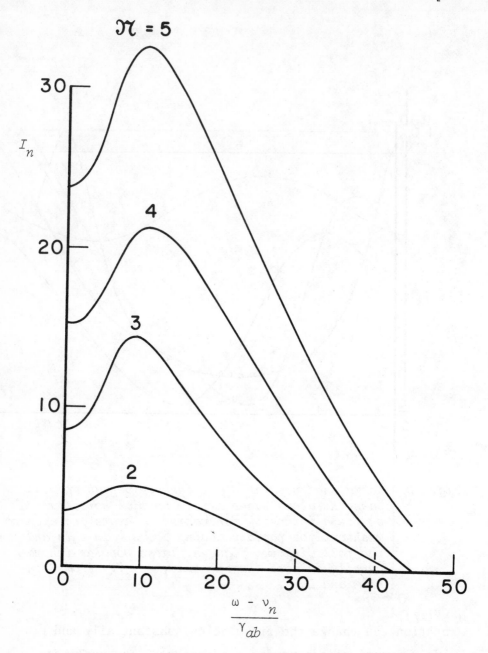

Fig. 13. *Dimensionless intensity vs. detuning for several*
values of relative excitation. Laser parameters
are normalized with respect to the decay constant
γ_{ab} *as follows:* $\gamma_a=0.6\gamma_{ab}$, $\gamma_b=1.4\gamma_{ab}$, $\gamma=\gamma_{ab}$,
$Ku=40\gamma_{ab}$. *From Stenholm and Lamb.*[8]

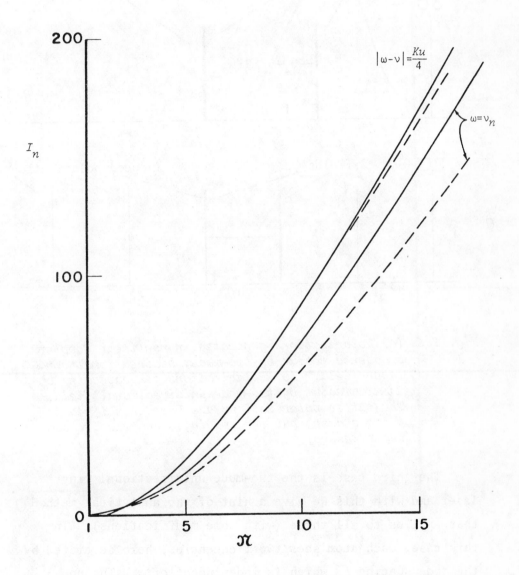

Fig. 14. *Laser intensity I_n vs. relative excitation for resonance ($\omega=\nu_n$) and for a detuning of Ku/4. The rate equation curves (dashed lines) show appreciable deviation from the exact (solid lines) for $I_n>10$ on resonance, but show good agreement for all intensities considered off line center. From Stenholm and Lamb.[8]*

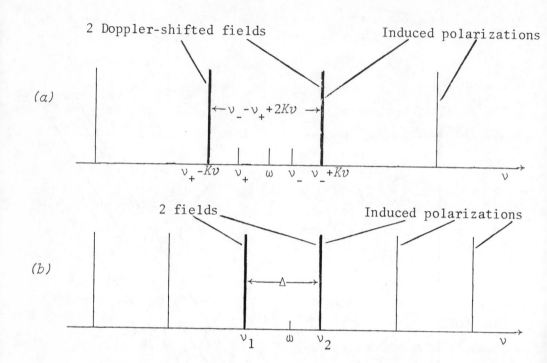

Fig. 15. (a) *Polarizations generated in nonlinear Doppler broadened medium by two-mode, bidirectional·ring laser field.* (b) *Polarizations generated in nonlinear medium by two-mode unidirectional field. The latter polarizations are Doppler shifted in the gas case, but the spacing* Δ *remains the same regardless of v.*

The third case is the two-mode unidirectional ring laser and with this we give a hint of the analytical method that applies to all three (with some modifications). In this case, each atom sees two frequencies, here separated by the mode spacing Δ, which is independent of v. The nonlinear medium beats as usual yielding an array of induced polarizations as depicted in Fig. 15b. Formally we represent this array by the Fourier series

$$p(z,\omega',t) = N(z,\omega',t) \sum_m p_m(\omega') \exp[-i(\nu_m t - K_m z)], \quad (44)$$

where $p_m(\omega')$ is a complex Fourier component at frequency ν_m. The population difference with its pulsations at integral multiples of Δ is given by

$$D(z,\omega',t) = N(z,\omega',t) \sum_{k=-\infty}^{\infty} d_k(\omega') \exp[ik(\Delta t - \pi z/L)].$$

$$(45)$$

Here the real Fourier coefficient d_0 is the dc saturated population difference given approximately by the REA method. The coefficient $d_k(\omega') = d_{-k}{}^*(\omega')$ corresponds to population pulsations at the frequency Δ.

We plug these Fourier series into medium equations of motion something like (9) and obtain algebraic equations for the d_k's. These, in turn, lead to a complex continued fraction

$$r_l = \frac{d_l}{d_{l-1}} = \frac{c_{-1,l}}{c_{0,l} + c_{1,l} r_{l+1}} \quad (46)$$

in which the complex constants c_{jl} are functions of the mode amplitudes and Lorentzians of various detunings. The complex polarization can be written in terms of the r_l, which, in turn, can be evaluated numerically on a computer. The method is inherently transcendental in the mode amplitudes and hence must be pursued on a fairly substantial machine. Our continued fraction differs from Stenholm and Lamb's,[8]

but we have reproduced their answers. In addition, our
program treats all three cases.

1-7. WHERE TO NOW?

In our discussion we have considered strong-signal
laser operation for one- and two-mode operation with rate
equation and "exact" methods, and media which are either
homogeneously or inhomogeneously broadened. The questions
arise as to what else one can consider and how generally
applicable the theories are.

Considering the first of these, note that multimode
mode-locked operation[†] is characterized by the mode frequency
condition

$$\nu_n = \nu_q + (n-q)\Delta, \tag{47}$$

where Δ is the intermode spacing. Hence the beat frequencies
between mode frequencies are all integral multiples of Δ,
just like the two-mode case! And therefore the approach of
Sec. 6 can be generalized to treat multimode modelocked
operation, a generalization I hope to publish with numerical
results before long. In this connection, the multimode,
standing-wave, *Doppler* broadened case is not so straightforward, for as we saw in Sec. 6, each atom sees two

---

[†]For further discussion of mode locking, see Chap. 9, Vol. 2
by Von der Linde and Chap. 2, Vol. 2 by Dienes.

frequencies, even for a *single* field mode. The multimode case is horrendous to say the least, and as yet I have not been able to reduce it to computational form.

With regard to the limitations of the theories, note that we have ignored transverse variations of the field and of the excitation mechanism, we have assumed high-Q, stable cavities, and we have supposed that the excitation mechanism varies little during atomic and cavity lifetimes. None of these assumptions is particularly valid for the TEA or GDL lasers (see Chap. 5), although they are quite good for typical operation of He-Ne and other reasonable lasers. Nevertheless the basic principles enter any laser device and with the understanding gained from the simple theories, one is in a better position to intuit the nature of operation of the next crazy laser to be invented.

ACKNOWLEDGEMENTS

I would like to thank Fred Aronowitz, V. P. Chebotayev, Jarel Hambenne, Fred Hopf, Willis Lamb and Stig Stenholm for helpful conversations. This work was supported in part by the Air Force Weapons Laboratory, Kirtland Air Force Base, Albuquerque, New Mexico.

APPENDIX

This appendix bridges the gap between the polarization and population variables of Eqs. (9a) - (9c) and the wave function $\psi(\vec{r},t)$ of quantum mechanics. The bridge consists of the density matrix ρ, which we define and give a simple interpretation for. A more complete development is given in Chaps. 1, 2 and 7 of Ref. 1.

The wave function $\psi(\vec{r},t)$ gives all knowable information about a system, say an electron in an atom. It is most easily interpreted in terms of its absolute value squared, $|\psi(\vec{r},t)|^2$, which is the *probability density* of finding the electron in the differential volume d^3r. In this interpretation, $\psi(\vec{r},t)$ is a probability density amplitude. Since the electron is somewhere, $\int d^3r |\psi(\vec{r},t)|^2 = 1$.

For the interaction of radiation with matter, it is convenient to write $\psi(\vec{r},t)$ in terms of energy eigenfunctions. Each of these functions has its own spatial distribution, the more spread out, the more energy (electron is not as deep on the average, in the electrostatic potential well). An arbitrary spatial function, e.g., $\psi(\vec{r},t)$ can be written in terms of these energy functions allowing us to watch how things change under the influence of light. Specifically transitions occur, that is to say, the superposition of energy eigenfunctions changes in time. The quantitative development is given by the Schrödinger equation

$$i\hbar\dot{\psi}(\vec{r},t) \;=\; H\psi(\vec{r},t) \tag{A1}$$

in which the Hamiltonian H is the energy operator for the system. For our purposes, H is the sum of the internal

energy of the atom, H_0, and the electric-dipole interaction
energy between the atom and the field, $-e\vec{r}\cdot\vec{E}$, that is,

$$H = H_0 - e\vec{r}\cdot\vec{E}. \tag{A2}$$

For simplicity, we suppose that the light interaction
is resonant for only two energy levels, labeled by a and b,
and hence that $\psi(\vec{r},t)$ can be written as the particular superposition

$$\psi(\vec{r},t) = c_a(t)u_a(\vec{r}) + c_b(t)u_b(\vec{r}). \tag{A3}$$

Here u_a and u_b are eigenfunctions of H_0 with eigenvalues $\hbar\omega_a$
and $\hbar\omega_b$ respectively. From the normalization property,
$|c_a|^2 + |c_b|^2 = 1$, and $|c_a|^2$ is the probability that the
atom is in the upper state. Plugging (A3) into (A1) and
using the orthonomality condition $\int d^3 r u_\alpha^*(\vec{r})u_\beta(\vec{r}) = \delta_{\alpha,\beta}$
($\alpha,\beta = a$ or b), we get the equations of motion for the
probability amplitudes c_a and c_b, namely,

$$i\hbar\,\dot{c}_a(t) = \hbar\omega_a c_a + V_{ab}c_b, \tag{A4}$$

$$i\hbar\,\dot{c}_b(t) = V_{ba}c_a + \hbar\omega_b c_b, \tag{A5}$$

where the matrix element $V_{ab} = V_{ba}^* = -\int d^3 r u_a^* e\vec{r}\cdot\vec{E}u_b = -\wp E$.
We have assumed that the interaction energy operator connects
only the levels a and b and has no effect on the energies of

the levels themselves. We further take the reduced electric-dipole matrix element to be real (without loss of generality).

We wish to know the polarization and populations of the medium. The polarization of an individual atom is given by the expectation value of $e\vec{r}$, that is,

$$\langle e\vec{r} \rangle = \int d^3r \; \psi^*(\vec{r},t) e\vec{r} \psi(\vec{r},t)$$

$$= \wp c_a c_b^* + \text{c.c.} \tag{A6}$$

This is just the average of the electric dipole over the electron distribution function $|\psi(\vec{r},t)|^2$. The polarization of the medium is proportional to this expectation value. Similarly, the populations are proportional to the probabilities $|c_a|^2$ and $|c_b|^2$. Hence we are primarily concerned not with c_a and c_b alone, but with the bilinear quantities, $c_a c_a^*$, $c_a c_b^*$, $c_b c_a^*$ and $c_b c_b^*$. These quantities are conveniently organized in matrix form as

$$\rho = \begin{pmatrix} c_a c_a^* & c_a c_b^* \\ c_b c_a^* & c_b c_b^* \end{pmatrix} = \begin{pmatrix} \rho_{aa} & \rho_{ab} \\ \rho_{ba} & \rho_{bb} \end{pmatrix} \tag{A7}$$

which is called a density matrix.

From the equations of motion (A4) and (A5) for the probability amplitudes, we see quite readily that the polarization component ρ_{ab} has the equation of motion

$$\dot{\rho}_{ab} = \dot{c}_a c_b^* + c_a \dot{c}_b^*$$

$$= -i\omega\rho_{ab} + \frac{i}{\hbar} V_{ab}[\rho_{aa} - \rho_{bb}], \tag{A8}$$

and the probabilities obey

$$\dot{\rho}_{aa} = -\frac{i}{\hbar} V_{ab}\rho_{ba} + \text{c.c.} \tag{A9}$$

$$\dot{\rho}_{bb} = +\frac{i}{\hbar} V_{ab}\rho_{ba} + \text{c.c.} \tag{A10}$$

The description of a laser medium is conveniently given in terms of averages over these single atom cases in which decay due to spontaneous emission and collisions are included along with pumping. Specifically, we define a "population" matrix

$$\rho(z,t) = \sum_{\alpha=a,b} \int_{-\infty}^{t} dt_o \lambda_\alpha(z,t_o)\rho(\alpha,z,t_o,t), \tag{A11}$$

where λ_α is the number of atoms/cm^3/sec pumped to the αth level and $\rho(\alpha,z,t_o,t)$ is the density matrix for a single atom excited to the αth level at time $t=t_o$ and place z. To understand the latter, note that by this definition,

$$\rho(\alpha,z,t_o,t=t_o) = \begin{pmatrix} \delta_{\alpha a} & 0 \\ 0 & \delta_{\alpha b} \end{pmatrix}.$$

As one can show by computing $\dot{\rho}(z,t)$, the matrix $\rho(z,t)$, too, has component equations of motion (A8) - (A10), but with λ_a appearing on the RHS of (A9) and λ_b on the RHS of (A10).

We further suppose that the decay of ρ_{aa} occurs at the rate $-\gamma_a \rho_{aa}$, the decay of ρ_{bb} goes at $-\gamma_b \rho_{bb}$, and the decay of ρ_{ab} at $-\gamma \rho_{ab}$. Here we ordinarily take $\gamma > \frac{1}{2}(\gamma_a + \gamma_b)$ since there are collisions that jilt the atomic dipole without changing the atom's energy. Combining these effects, we obtain

$$\dot{\rho}_{ab}(z,t) = -(i\omega+\gamma)\rho_{ab} + \frac{i}{\hbar} V_{ab}\left[\rho_{aa}(z,t) - \rho_{bb}(z,t)\right],$$

(A12)

$$\dot{\rho}_{aa}(z,t) = \lambda_a - \gamma_a \rho_{aa}(z,t) - \left[\frac{i}{\hbar} V_{ab}\rho_{ba}(z,t) + \text{c.c.}\right],$$

(A13)

$$\dot{\rho}_{bb}(z,t) = \lambda_b - \gamma_b \rho_{bb}(z,t) + \left[\frac{i}{\hbar} V_{ab}\rho_{ba}(z,t) + \text{c.c.}\right].$$

(A14)

The polarization and population equations of motion (9) are given by (A12) - (A14) with the definitions $p \equiv \rho_{ab}(z,t)$ and $N_\alpha \equiv \rho_{\alpha\alpha}(z,t)$.

REFERENCES

1. M. Sargent III, M. O Scully, and W. E. Lamb, Jr., *Laser Physics*, Addison-Wesley, Reading, Mass. (1974).

2. M. Sargent III, *Appl. Phys.* **1**, 133 (1973).

3. W. R. Bennett, Jr., in *Brandeis Summer Institute in Theoretical Physics (1969)*, Gordon and Breach, New York (1972).

4. W. E. Lamb, Jr., *Phys. Rev.* 134, A1429 (1964).

5. J. L. Hall, in *Atomic Physics* 3, S. J. Smith and D. K. Walters, eds., Plenum Press, New York, p. 615 (1973). See also Chap. 10, Vol. 2 by K. Evenson.

6. R. G. Brewer, *Science* 178, 247 (1972). See also Chap. 12, Vol. 2 by R. Shoemaker.

7. M. Lax, in *Brandeis Summer Institute in Theoretical Physics (1966)*, Gordon and Breach, New York (1968).

8. S. Stenholm and W. E. Lamb, Jr., *Phys. Rev.* 181, 618 (1969).

9. B. J. Feldman and M. Feld, *Phys. Rev.* A1, 1375 (1970).

10. H. K. Holt, *Phys. Rev.* A2, 233 (1970).

11. L. Menegozzi and W. E. Lamb, Jr., *Phys. Rev.* A8, 2103 (1973).

12. J. Hambenne and M. Sargent III, to be published. The material in Sec. 6 was presented at the Spring 1973 Meeting of the Optical Society of America [M. Sargent III, *J. Opt. Soc. Am.* 63, 503 (1973)]. See also M. Salomaa and R. Salomaa, *Physica Fennica* 8, 289 (1973).

A PRELIMINARY ACCOUNT OF A
NEW APPROACH TO UNSTABLE RESONATORS

Hansen Shih, Marlan O. Scully

Stephen F. Jacobs

2.1.   INTRODUCTION

Unstable resonators are of practical interest because
their large interaction volume is essential for high power
lasers, because they avoid the problem of mirror damage,
and because they serve as a means to achieve mode control.[1,2]
Although intensity distributions and diffraction losses
have been shown to be calculable for specific cases,[3] there
have as yet been no satisfactory theoretical derivations of
the mode structures in unstable resonators. The present
approach is a multimode analysis of the problem which includes effects of an active medium. It is of interest to
note that a similar problem (in the sense that it involved
a very complicated multi-mode analysis) has been treated
elsewhere and provides encouragement and moral support for
the present approach.[4] Using this picture, we are able to
describe intensity distributions, diffraction loss and mode
frequencies continuously as the resonator configuration is
varied from stable to unstable. Although the preliminary

results are idealized and as yet untested, we believe that
the physical insight we have already gained, in the form
analogies with magnetism, will lead to the synthesis of improved designs and will facilitate analysis of factors
which degrade resonator beam quality.

Using simple geometrical optics arguments, it was
demonstrated[1] that the output coupling ratio of the lowest
order mode in an unstable resonator is essentially independent of the Fresnel number (or mirror size). It then seemed
meaningful to discuss the limiting cases of unstable cavities with infinitely large Fresnel numbers, for which analytical solutions were easily found.[2,5-7] The unstable modes
were simply the analytical continuation of the modes from
the stable region.[6] However, they do not converge in the
transverse directions and therefore can hardly be regarded
as physical solutions.

Another often used approach has been to calculate
numerically the "self-consistent fields" in very much the
same way as for a stable resonator.[2,8,9] The lowest order
modes are shown to be more or less uniformly distributed in
the cavity bounded by the mirrors, whereas the modes with
higher order symmetries are shifted more toward the mirror
edges.

In both approaches mentioned above the "modes" have
been frequently considered only for empty cavities. In
other words, the effects of gains and losses of the lasing
media on the mode structures have often been neglected.

In this paper we present a different approach in which
the modes for unstable resonators are constructed as super-
positions of the known modes of some conveniently chosen
stable resonator. Both the temporal and spatial behaviors

are inherently included in the theory, and an extension to
cover the case of nonlinear interactions is clearly indicated. Physically, this is realized by considering the unstable cavity to be equivalent to a conveniently chosen
stable cavity, made unstable by the introduction of concave
lens (Sec. 2.2). The lens serves as a mode coupler (Sec.
2.3.), with its inverse focal length the coupling parameter.
Having shown how the introduction of a lens (resonator
going unstable) mixes the modes to build a new set of modes
which satisfy the boundary conditions, we can represent the
lens effect as a driving polarization term in the wave
equation (Sec. 2.4.). This done, it is a straightforward
matter to introduce the effect of the lasing atoms via addition of further polarization terms which can include both
linear and nonlinear interactions.

Diffraction loss is simulated by injecting an appropriate amount of resonant atoms uniformly into the concave
lens. In other words, we let the lens dielectric susceptibility become complex. It is planned to treat the effects
of the atoms and nonlinear mode coupling in a later paper.
The object of the present analysis is to establish the
feasibility of handling the unstable resonator problem via
the present multi-mode approach, including the effects of
an active medium in a natural way. One of the successes of
the present theory is that mode behavior may be studied continuously through the transition region between stable and
unstable operation.

2.2. EQUIVALENT RESONATORS

Figure 1a depicts the type of unstable optical resonator we are going to investigate. It has length D' and is bounded at its two ends by mirrors M_1' and M_2' with radius of curvature R_1' and R_2' respectively. Stability of the resonator is characterized by the parameter g' defined as,[10]

$$g' = \left(1 - \frac{D'}{R_1'}\right)\left(1 - \frac{D'}{R_2'}\right). \tag{1}$$

It is unstable if $g' > 1$ or $g' < 0$.

Instead of this resonator, let us consider the equivalent system in Fig. 1b which has a concave lens L inserted between the end mirrors M_1 and M_2. Without the lens, the cavity is chosen to be stable, i.e.,

$$0 \leq g = \left(1 - \frac{D}{R_1}\right)\left(1 - \frac{D}{R_2}\right) \leq 1.$$

For this resonator the modes are well known.[10]

We take $R_1 = R_1'$, $D = D'$ and assume that the lens L lies very close to M_2. The combination of L and M_2 is assumed to have focal length equivalent to that of M_2'. This can be realized if we take

$$\frac{1}{f} = \frac{1}{R_2'} - \frac{1}{R_2},$$

where f denotes the focal length of the lens L.

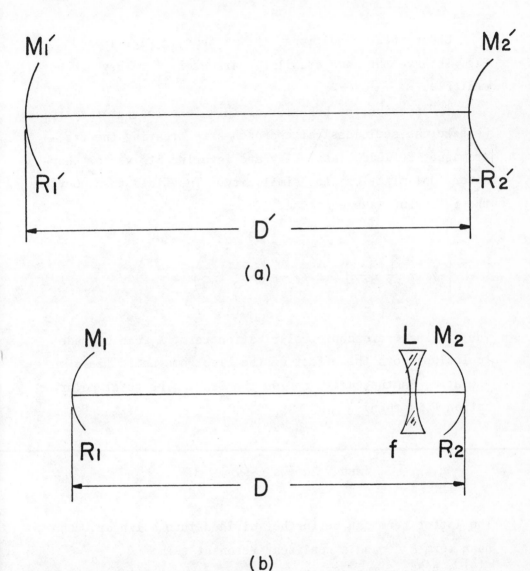

Fig. 1. *(a) Schematic diagram for an unstable optical resonator. (b) Stable resonator with a diverging lens inserted is optically equivalent to the unstable system in (a).*

Under these conditions, the systems in Fig. 1a and
Fig. 1b have the same stability parameter g'. They are both
unstable.

To describe the behavior of this lens-resonator system,
we take the semiclassical approach here treating the electromagnetic field classically and ignoring its vector character (polarization) for simplicity. The field then obeys
the following wave equation,

$$\left[-\nabla^2 + \frac{1}{c^2} \frac{\partial^2}{\partial t^2} \right] E(\vec{r}, t) = -\mu_o \left(\frac{\partial}{\partial t} \right)^2 P(\vec{r}, t). \tag{2}$$

The driving macroscopic polarization term, P, can be made
to include both the effect of the electromagnetic field on
the atoms in the cavity and on the lens. The total polarization P is then

$$P = P_{lens} + P_{atoms}.$$

The latter term can be further divided into a linear, resonant term $P^{(L)}$ and a nonlinear resonant term: $P_{atoms} =$
$P^{(L)} + P^{(NL)}_{res}$. The effect of the nonresonant $P^{(L)}$ is to
change the velocity of light from c to v. To treat the resonant contributions we can use the simple model of quantum
mechanical two-level atoms interacting with the classical
electromagnetic field.[11] Separating the linear and nonlin-
ear effects and denoting them by $P^{(L)}_{res}$ and P^{NL}_{res}, respectively,
the wave equation becomes

$$\left[-\nabla^2 + \frac{1}{v^2}\frac{\partial^2}{\partial t^2}\right]E = -\mu_o\left(\frac{\partial}{\partial t}\right)^2\left[P_{res}^{(L)} + P_{res}^{NL} + P_{lens}\right], \quad (3)$$

where

$$P_{lens} = \begin{cases} \varepsilon_0\chi E & \textit{inside the lens} \\ \\ 0 & \textit{elsewhere} \end{cases} \quad (4)$$

In the present paper we neglect effects nonlinear in the electric field and thus drop the term P_{res}^{NL}.

Suppose now that, for the electric field E as well as the polarization P, the time and spatial dependence is separable in the sense that we may write

$$E(\vec{r},t) = Re\left[\sum_\xi E_\xi(t)\mu_\xi(\vec{r})\right]$$

$$\quad (5)$$

$$P(\vec{r},t) = Re\left[\sum_\xi P_\xi(t)\mu_\xi(\vec{r})\right],$$

where we let $\{\mu_\xi\}$ be a complete set of orthogonal eigensolutions satisfying

$$\nabla^2\mu_\xi = -(2\pi/\lambda_\xi)^2\,\mu_\xi,$$

and the boundary conditions be those imposed by the mirrors in the system of Fig. 1b with the lens removed.

From the orthonormality condition,

$$\int_{\text{Cavity}} d^3r\mu_{\xi*}(\vec{r})\mu_{\xi'}(\vec{r}) = \delta_{\xi\xi'} \, ,$$

and the assumption that the field amplitudes and phases vary little in an optical wavelength (slowly varying approximation),[9] the wave equation of (3) reduces to a set of coupled first-order time-dependent equations

$$\left[\frac{\partial}{\partial t} + i\omega_\xi\right] E_\xi(t) = i \frac{\omega_\xi}{2} v^2\mu_0 P_\xi(t), \tag{6}$$

where

$$\omega_\xi = 2\pi v/\lambda_\xi.$$

If we further assume that the laser field inside the cavity consists of mixings of high-Q modes, the diffraction loss can be incorporated into our equation as phenomenological damping $\Gamma_\xi^{(d)}$.

$$\left[\frac{\partial}{\partial t} + i\omega_\xi\left(1 - \tfrac{1}{2}\chi_\xi^L\right) + \Gamma_\xi^{(d)}\right] E_\xi(t)$$

$$= \sum_{\xi'\neq\xi}\left\{i \frac{\omega_\xi}{2} \chi_{\xi\xi'}^L E_{\xi'}(t) + i \frac{\omega_\xi}{2} v^2\mu_0 P_\xi^{res}\right\} \tag{7}$$

where

$$\chi_{\xi\xi'}^{L} = \frac{v^2}{c^2} \int_{\text{lens}} d^3r \mu_{\xi*}(\vec{r}) \chi \mu_{\xi'}(\vec{r}),$$

(8)

and

$$\chi_{\xi}^{L} = \chi_{\xi\xi'}^{L}.$$

(9)

2.3. THE LENS EFFECT

Let the mirrors M_1, M_2 and the lens L in Fig. 1b be bounded by spherical surfaces so that the system is symmetric about the z-axis. It is then natural to solve the equation,

$$\left[\nabla^2 + \left(\frac{2\pi}{\lambda_\xi} \right)^2 \right] \mu_\xi = 0$$

in cylindrical coordinates (z, r, ϕ) where r denotes the distance from the z-axis and ϕ the azimuth angle.

Replacing the mode numbers ξ by (q, ℓ, m) and using the slowly varying amplitude approximation, gives

$$\mu_{q\ell m} = C_{q\ell m} \frac{1}{w} e^{-im\phi} \left\{ \tilde{r}^m L_\ell^m(\tilde{r}^2) \exp[-\tilde{r}^2/2] \right\}$$

$$\times \exp\left[-i \frac{2\pi}{\lambda} z - i \frac{2}{\tilde{R}} \frac{r^2}{w_o^2} \right.$$

$$\left. + i(2\ell + m + 1) \tan^{-1} \tilde{z} \right],$$

(10)

where z is measured from the beam waist, and

$$\tilde{r}^2 = 2r^2/w^2$$

$$w = w_0\sqrt{1 + \tilde{z}^2}$$

$$\tilde{z} = z/\left((w_0^2/\lambda)\pi\right)$$

$$\tilde{R} = \tilde{z} + \tilde{z}^{-1},$$

L_ℓ^m is an associated Laguerre polynomial,

$$L_\ell^m(\chi) = \sum_{m=0}^{\ell} (-1)^{m'} \binom{\ell+m}{\ell-m'} \frac{1}{m'!} \chi^{m'}$$

and $C_{q\ell m}$ is the normalization constant.

For perfect mirrors M_1, M_2, the boundary condition that $\mu_{q\ell m}$ vanishes at the two mirror surfaces restricts the wavelength λ to discrete values specified by

$$1/\lambda = (1/2D)[(q+1) + (2\ell + m + 1)\tfrac{\theta}{2}] \qquad (11)$$

$$\theta = (2/\pi)\cos^{-1}\sqrt{[1 - (D/R_1)][1 - (D/R_2)]}, \qquad (12)$$

where q, ℓ, m are integers.

Once λ is specified, the minimum beam width w_0 is determined by

$$w_0^2/\lambda = \frac{\sqrt{D(R_1+R_2-D)(R_1-D)(R_2-D)}}{R_1+R_2-2D} \equiv L_c(R_1,R_2,D). \, (13)$$

For a thin lens L, its longitudinal dimension is negligible compared to its radius of curvature R_L. We then take, for the lens L centered at z_L, the susceptibility to be

$$
\chi_L(\vec{r}) \; \simeq \; \begin{cases} \chi & \text{if } |z-z_L| < \dfrac{r^2}{2R_L} \\[2ex] 0 & \text{elsewhere.} \end{cases} \tag{14}
$$

For simplicity let us assume a "short cavity" inside through which the beam width w is essentially constant, i.e.,

$$
D \; << \; L_c \; = \; \pi w_o^2 / \lambda .
$$

We further let the susceptibility χ and the radius of curvature R_L of the lens approach infinity, but keep their ratio constant. The dioptric power f^{-1} of the lens $(f^{-1} = -\chi/R_L)$ thus remains unchanged.

For laser oscillation, we only have to consider the mixing of modes with small fractional differences in the wavelength. With these assumptions and use of recurrence and orthonormality properties of the Laguerre polynomials, we obtain

$$
\chi^L_{q\ell m, q'\ell'm'} \; = \; f^{-1} \frac{w^2}{D} \, \delta_{mm'} \Big\{ \delta_{\ell\ell'} \, (2\ell+m+1)
$$

$$
- \delta_{\ell+\ell'} \, \sqrt{(\ell+1)(\ell+m+1)} \; \exp[-2i \, \tan^{-1}\hat{z}]
$$

$$
- \delta_{\ell-1,\ell'} \, \sqrt{\ell(\ell+m)} \; \exp[+2i \, \tan^{-1}\hat{z}] \Big\} . \tag{15}
$$

For the resonators with the special symmetries which
we are considering, Eq. (15) implies that there is no
mixing among modes with different azimuth mode-number m's
and that if we regard the modes with the same mode numbers
(m, ℓ) as a single "particle," the interaction among them
may then be depicted as a linear chain consisting of these
particles with nearest neighbor interactions.

2.4.   RESONANT POLARIZATION

For the resonant contribution to the polarization, the
medium may be adequately described by a system of two-level
atoms. The energy difference $\hbar\omega_0$ between the upper and
lower levels (a and b) of a single atom is approximately
the same as the photon energy $\hbar\omega$ of the cavity laser field.
We neglect the effects of inhomogeneous broadening and
assume that the atomic collisions can be summarized phenom-
enologically by decay constants γ_a and γ_b for the upper and
lower levels respectively. Using the equations of motion
for the density matrix of the atomic system, we can obtain
the solutions for the polarization by well-known techniques.[11]

For simplicity, let us consider the single-mode case
so that we can write

$$E(\vec{r}, t) = \mathrm{Re}\left[A_\xi(t) e^{-i\omega_\xi t} \mu_\xi(\vec{r})\right].$$

In the rotating wave approximation we then have the following expression for the polarization:

$$\langle P_{res}\rangle = \mathrm{Re}\left\{\frac{-i/\hbar |ex_{ab}|^2}{i\Delta\omega_\xi + \gamma_{ab}} \frac{1}{1-R_\xi} [\Delta N(r)]\right.$$

$$\left. \times \left[A_\xi(t) exp(-i\omega_\xi t)\mu_\xi(r)\right]\right\} , \quad (16)$$

and

$$R_\xi = 2(i/\hbar)^2 |ex_{ab}A_\xi\mu_\xi|^2 \frac{1}{\gamma} \mathrm{Re}\left(\frac{2}{i\Delta\omega_\xi + \gamma_{ab}}\right), \quad (17)$$

where

$$[\Delta N(\vec{r})] = \frac{\lambda_a(\vec{r})}{\gamma_a} - \frac{\lambda_b(\vec{r})}{\gamma_b}$$

$$\gamma^{-1} = \gamma_a^{-1} + \gamma_b^{-1}$$

$$\Delta\omega_\xi = \omega_0 - \omega_\xi$$

$$ex_{ab} = e\langle a|x|b\rangle,$$

and λ_a and λ_b are the pumping rates into the upper and lower levels respectively.

In general, the laser field E consists of many modes, i.e.,

$$E(\vec{r}, t) \;=\; \text{Re} \sum_{\xi} exp(-i\omega_{\xi} t) A_{\xi}(t) \mu_{\xi}(\vec{r}).$$

Equations (16) and (17) can easily be generalized to cover this situation.

In the weak field limit, the linear approximation is valid. We have

$$\langle P_{res} \rangle \;=\; \text{Re} \sum_{\xi} \chi_{res}^{(L)}(\vec{r}) exp(-i\omega_{\xi} t) A_{\xi}(t) \mu_{\xi}(\vec{r})$$

and

$$\chi_{res}^{(L)}(\vec{r}) \;=\; \frac{i}{\hbar} |ex_{ab}|^2 \frac{1}{i\Delta\omega_{\xi} + \gamma_{ab}} [\Delta N(\vec{r})]. \tag{18}$$

In compliance with Eq. (5), we see

$$P_{\xi}^{res}(t) \;\simeq\; \sum_{\xi} \varepsilon_0 \left(\chi_{res}^{(L)} \right)_{\xi\xi'} E_{\xi'}(t), \tag{19}$$

where

$$\left(\chi_{res}^{(L)} \right)_{\xi\xi'} \;=\; 1/\varepsilon_0 (-i/\hbar) |ex_{ab}|^2 \frac{1}{i\Delta\omega_{\xi'} + \gamma_{ab}}$$

$$\times \int_{cavity} d^3r \mu_{\xi}^*(\vec{r}) [\Delta N(\vec{r})] \mu_{\xi'}(r).$$

If the pumping is uniform, ΔN is constant inside the cavity, and it follows that $(\chi_{res})_{\xi\xi'}$ is then diagonal

$$(\chi_{res})_{\xi\xi} = \left[(-i/\hbar) \; 1/\varepsilon_0 \; |ex_{ab}|^2 \; \frac{(\Delta N)}{i\Delta\omega_\xi + \gamma_{ab}} \right] \delta_{\xi\xi'}. \tag{20}$$

Consequently there is no mixing among different ξ-modes due to the resonant effect.

Neglecting small changes in the phase velocity v, we find that Eq. (7) becomes,

$$\left[\frac{\partial}{\partial t} + i\omega_\xi (1 - \tfrac{1}{2}\chi_\xi^L) + \Gamma_\xi \right] E_\xi(t) = \sum_{\xi' \neq \xi} i \, \frac{\omega_\xi}{2} \, \chi_{\xi\xi'}^L E_{\xi'}(t), \tag{21}$$

where

$$\Gamma_\xi \cong \Gamma_\xi^{(d)} + \frac{\omega_\xi}{2} \left(\frac{v}{c}\right)^2 \frac{|ex_{ab}|^2}{\varepsilon_0 \hbar} \frac{(\Delta N)\gamma_{ab}}{(\Delta\omega_\xi)^2 + \gamma_{ab}^2} .$$

Therefore we see that, under the assumption of uniform pumping, it is solely the presence of the lens which mixes the different ξ-modes in first order.

2.5. OVERVIEW

Because the details of this treatment are published elsewhere[22] and may not be of interest here, we present below only an outline of the treatment. We see that the wave equation in the form (21) can be written in a Schrödinger-equation-like form

$$i\hbar \frac{\partial}{\partial t} E(t) = (H_0 + H') E(t).$$

It is shown that for resonators with cylindrical symmetry, there is no mixing among modes with different azimuthal number m, and we therefore confine ourselves for simplicity to the case $m = 0$. If we regard the modes with the same mode numbers (m, ℓ) as a single "particle," the interaction among them may be depicted as a linear chain consisting of these particles with only nearest neighbor interactions H'.

The Lens Effect is then treated by perturbation theory (see Appendix), neglecting resonant contributions and losses. It is shown that, as the resonator goes from stable to unstable, the linear mode mixing coefficients behave like the magnetic susceptibility near the ferromagnetic-diamagnetic phase transition, with θ, Eq. (11), playing the role of temperature.

To investigate mode behavior in the unstable region it becomes necessary to go beyond the perturbation treatment to a strong coupling theory. We choose to construct the unstable resonator modes out of known modes in a marginally stable resonator (near $\theta = 0$). We show that we are then dealing with modes where the frequency differences between adjacent axial modes (q) is much larger than those between adjacent transverse modes (ℓ). Another simplification comes about by further assuming that the resonant linewidth γ is wide compared with the frequency spacing between adjacent transverse modes, yet much narrower than that between adjacent axial modes. The lowest order transverse mode is

taken to be in exact resonance with the lasing atoms as
indicated in Fig. 2.

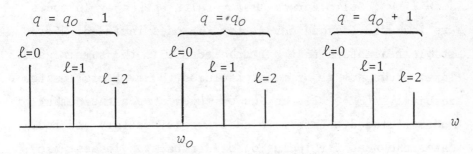

*Fig. 2.   Lowest-order mode of (q_0) is chosen to be at
atomic line center.*

We can therefore ignore coupling of modes with different
axial number q. This simplification, along with the fact
that axial symmetry prevents coupling of modes with different azimuth number m, reduces the general problem of three-
dimensional coupling (involving mode-numbers q,ℓ,m) to that
of a one-dimensional coupling, involving ℓ only. As shown
previously, this has only nearest-neighbor interactions.

A stability parameter is defined to be

$$F = \frac{f\lambda_0\theta}{2W^2} \approx \frac{f}{R}$$

and it is seen that

$$0 < F < 1 \qquad \text{is unstable}$$

$$F = 0,1 \qquad \text{is marginally stable}$$

$$\left.\begin{array}{l} F > 1 \\ \\ F < 0 \end{array}\right\} \quad \text{is stable.}$$

Figure 3 shows the numerical results: Field amplitude vs. normalized radial distance for various degrees of resonator stability. Solid curves show results when only 10 modes are included; dashed curves for 20 modes included. For stable resonators ($F^{-1} < 1$) the result is the same regardless of the number of modes included, however, for unstable resonators ($F^{-1} > 1$) the answer depends upon the number of modes included. This is clearly unsatisfactory and indicates the need for inclusion of diffraction losses which, in a real situation, serve to limit the number of higher-order modes that can build up. Figure 4 shows the results of introduction of simulated diffraction loss via an absorbing concave lens. All curves are given for the marginally stable case $F^{-1} = 1$, with varying amounts of loss. It is seen that as losses increase the inclusion of additional modes ceases to affect the mode pattern. This is a satisfying result.

Finally, it is shown in Ref. 20, that the numerical results above can be understood analytically by an asymptotic theory where the number of coupled modes goes to infinity. Linewidths and mode frequencies are also included in the theory.

In summary, we have devised a new analytical method to describe the mode structure of unstable laser oscillators. The treatment can take into account both linear and nonlinear effects of the gain medium. Uniform loss is easily included, while diffraction loss has been simulated by introducing radially increasing absorption at the mirrors. This simulation will require modification for sharp-edged mirrors, but corresponds quite well to mirrors whose edge reflectivity is tapered.[16-21]

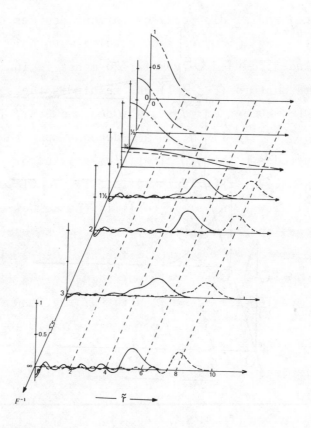

Fig. 3. *Mode pattern for the lowest eigenfrequency mode.*
Vertical axis is the field amplitude $\bar{u}_L{}^0$, horizon-
tal axis denotes the normalized radial distance $\vec{r}$ =
$\sqrt{2}(r/w)$, and the third dimension indicates the
stability parameter F^{-1}. Solid curves are for
ℓ_{max} = 10, and dashed curves for ℓ_{max} = 20. Abrupt
changes in mode pattern near the transition F^{-1} is
observed.

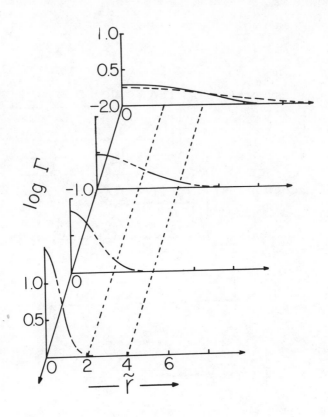

Fig. 4. *The lowest-order mode patterns in the marginal case $F^{-1} = 1$. The field amplitudes $\bar{\mu}_L{}^0$ are shown for various loss parameters, $\Gamma = 10^{-2}$, 10^{-1}, 1, 10. Solid curves are for $\ell_{max} = 10$ while the dashed curves for $\ell_{max} = 20$. Except for the case $\Gamma = 0$, the results for $\ell_{max} = 10$ and 20 are almost indistinguishable here.*

By combining symmetry considerations with the assumption of sharp atomic resonance we have reduced a complicated three-dimensional problem to a much simpler one-dimensional linear chain problem, which we are able to solve in the asymptotic limit of an infinite number of coupled modes. Our asymptotic theory yields analytic solutions which describe well the temporal and spatial behavior of the lowest-loss resonant modes in unstable resonators, and these solutions agree with numerical computations. In the unstable as well as stable region the lowest-order mode pattern retains its Gaussian form when diffraction losses are simulated. Without losses, the beam diverges at the transition point ($F^{-1} = 1$); with loss included, the beam width remains finite.

ACKNOWLEDGMENTS

The authors would like to take this opportunity to acknowledge many stimulating discussions with Petras V. Avizonis.

This work was supported by the Air Force Weapons Laboratory, Kirtland Air Force Base, New Mexico.

APPENDIX

PERTURBATION TREATMENT

We here give a perturbation treatment on mode mixing. Since there is no mixing among modes with different azimuth mode-number m, we confine ourselves for simplicity, to the symmetric case $m = 0$. We also neglect the resonant, as well as diffractional, contributions for the present. We see that Eq. (21) can be written in a Schrödinger equation-like form as follows[†]

$$i\hbar \frac{\partial}{\partial t} |E(t)> = (\mathcal{H}_o + \mathcal{H}') |E(t)> . \tag{A1}$$

With $m = 0$, each of the "basis functions" of Eq. (A1) is represented by an axis whose direction is indicated by a unit vector $|q\ell>$ in the present Hilbert space. The component of the $|E>$ projection into each such axis is,

$$<q\ell|E> = E_{q,\ell}(t),$$

where $E_{q,\ell}$ is the expansion coefficient defined by Eq. (5) with $\xi \to (q,\ell,m=0)$.

With the help of Eq. (15), we obtain the following explicit expression for the matrix representation of the

---

[†]This is the wave equation in the Schrödinger picture. It is also referred to as the Heisenberg matrix equation.

unperturbed as well as the perturbing "Hamiltonians" $\mathcal{H}_o$ and $\mathcal{H}'$ respectively,

$$\langle q'\ell' | \mathcal{H}_o | q\ell \rangle = \delta_{qq'} \delta_{\ell\ell'} H^o_{q\ell} \tag{A2}$$

$$H^o_{q\ell} = \hbar\Omega_D [(q+1) + \ell\theta]$$

and

$$(q'\ell' | \mathcal{H}' | q\ell) = H'^{(+1)}_{q,\ell} \delta_{\ell+1,\ell'} + H'^{(0)}_{q\ell} \delta_{\ell,\ell'} + H'^{(-1)}_{q,\ell} \delta_{\ell-1,\ell'}$$

$$H'^{(\pm 1)}_{q,\ell} = \frac{W^2}{(-f)2\lambda} \left[\frac{\hbar\Omega_D}{2} \right] (\ell + \tfrac{1}{2} \pm \tfrac{1}{2}) e^{i\phi_L}$$

$$H'^{(0)}_{q,\ell} = \frac{W^2}{(-f)2\lambda} \left[\frac{\hbar\Omega_D}{2} \right] (2\ell + 1), \quad . \tag{A3}$$

where

$$\Omega_D = \pi v / D. \tag{A4}$$

We have assumed that there are only small fractional changes in the longitudinal number q, i.e.,

$$\left| \frac{q'-q}{q} \right| \ll 1.$$

We may therefore directly apply the time-independent perturbation theory of elementary quantum mechanics to our problem. It is obvious that in the weak-lens limit $(f^{-1} \to 0)$ we have

$$\left| \frac{H'^{(\pm 1)}_{q,\ell}}{H^O_{q\ell} - H^O_{q'\ell'}} \right| \ll 1$$

or

$$\left| \frac{W^2}{2f\lambda} \right| \ll \frac{q + \ell\theta}{q} \sim 1. \tag{A5}$$

The new eigenfunction $\mu_{q,\ell}(\underline{r})$ in the "perturbed" resonator-lens system of Fig. (1b) becomes

$$\mu_{q,\ell}(\underline{r}) \cong C_{q,\ell} \left\{ \mu_{q,\ell} + \frac{1}{(-f)} \sum_{q'} \left[e^{-i\phi_L} M_\ell^{(+1)}(q,q') \right. \right.$$

$$\left. \mu_{q',\ell+1} + e^{i\phi_L} M_\ell^{(-1)}(q,q')\mu_{q,\ell-1} \right]$$

$$\left. + \frac{1}{(-f)} \sum_{q'\neq q} M_\ell^{(0)}(q,q')\mu_{q',\ell} \right\}, \tag{A6}$$

where

$$\mu_{q,\ell} = \left. \mu_{q,\ell,m} \right|_{m=0}$$

$$C_{q,\ell} = \left[\int_{\text{cavity}} d^3r \left| \mu_{q,\ell} \right|^2 \right]^{-\frac{1}{2}}$$

and the "linear mixing coefficients" $M_\ell^{\Delta\ell}(q,q')$ are defined as:

$$M_\ell^{\Delta\ell}(q,q') = \begin{cases} \dfrac{\ell+1}{(q-q')-\theta} \times \dfrac{1}{2} \, (W^2/2\lambda) & \text{for } \Delta\ell = 1 \\[3ex] \dfrac{\ell}{(q-q')+\theta} \times \dfrac{1}{2} \, (W^2/2\lambda) & \text{for } \Delta\ell = -1 \\[3ex] \dfrac{-(2\ell+1)}{q-q'} \times \dfrac{1}{2} \, (W^2/2\lambda) & \text{for } \Delta\ell = 0 \\[3ex] 0 & \text{otherwise} \end{cases}$$

$$(A7)$$

Furthermore, the perturbed eigenfrequencies are found to be

$$(A8)$$

$$\Omega_{q,\ell} = \Omega_D \left\{ \left[(q+1) + \ell\theta \right] + \frac{1}{(-f)} \sum_{q'} \left[(\ell+1) M_\ell^{(+1)}(q,q') \right. \right.$$

$$\left. \left. + \ell M_\ell^{(-1)}(q,q') \right] - \frac{1}{(-f)} \sum_{q' \neq q} (2\ell+1) M_\ell^{(0)}(q,q') \right\} .$$

Recall that our discussions are based on the use of the mode functions and their associated frequencies for stable cavities. For such cavities the following inequality holds:

$$0 \; < \; \left(1 - \frac{D}{R_1}\right)\left(1 - \frac{D}{R_2}\right) \; < \; 1.$$

Correspondingly, the values of θ are restricted, through Eq. (12) to obey

$$1 \; > \; \theta \; > \; 0.$$

Near $\theta = 1$, $M_{\ell}^{+1}(q,q-1)$ and $M_{\ell}^{-1}(q,q+1)$ become very large and mode (q,ℓ) is strongly coupled to both modes $(q+1,\ell-1)$ and $(q-1,\ell+1)$. These terms dominate in the summation of Eq. (A6). We thus have approximately,

$$\mu_{q\ell} \; \cong \; C_{q\ell}\left\{\mu_{q\ell} + f^{-1}\left[e^{-i\phi_L} M_{\ell}^{+1}(q,q-1)\mu_{q-1,\ell+1}\right.\right.$$

$$\left.\left. + \; e^{i\phi_L} M_{\ell}^{-1}(q,q+1)\mu_{q+1,\ell-1}\right]\right\} \tag{A9}$$

for $1 - \theta \ll 1$.

On the other hand, near $\theta = 0$, $M_{\ell}^{+1}(q,q)$ and $M_{\ell}^{-1}(q,q)$ dominate and the mode (q,ℓ) is coupled strongly to modes $(q,\ell-1)$ and $(q,\ell+1)$. We have in the weak perturbation limit $f^{-1} \to 0$,

$$\mu_{q,\ell} \approx C_{q\ell} \left\{ \mu_q + f^{-1} \left[e^{-i\phi_L} M_\ell^{+1}(q,q) \mu_{q,\ell+1} \right. \right.$$

$$\left. \left. + e^{i\phi_L} M_\ell^{-1}(q,q) \mu_{q,\ell-1} \right] \right\} \tag{A10}$$

for $\theta \ll 1$.

The divergent behavior of the linear mixing coefficients is clearly indicated in the following expressions as we approach the transition region $\theta \approx 1$ or $\theta \approx 0$:

$$M_\ell^{\pm 1}(q, q\mp 1) = (\pm) \frac{\frac{1}{2}(\ell + \frac{1}{2} \pm \frac{1}{2})}{1-\theta} \left[\frac{W^2}{2\lambda} \right]$$

$$M_\ell^{\pm 1}(q, q) = (\mp) \frac{\frac{1}{2}(\ell + \frac{1}{2} \pm \frac{1}{2})}{\theta} \left[\frac{W^2}{2\lambda} \right]. \tag{A11}$$

Their behaviors near the transition resemble that, say, of the magnetic susceptibility near the Ferromagnetic-diamagnetic phase transition, with θ playing the role of temperature T. The analogous "Curie temperature" here is $\theta_c = 1$ for $M_\ell^{\pm 1}(q, q\pm 1)$, or $\theta_c = 0$ for $M_\ell^{\pm 1}(q, q)$.

REFERENCES

1. A. E. Siegman, *Proc. IEEE* 53, 277 (1965).

2. A. E. Siegman and R. Arrathoon, *IEEE J. Quant. Elect.*
    QE-3, 156 (1967).

3. R. J. Freiberg, P. P. Chenausky, and C. J. Buczek, *IEEE
    J. Quant. Elect.* QE-9, 716 (1973).

4. R. Lang, M. O. Scully, and W. E. Lamb, Jr., *Phys. Rev.
    A* 7, 1788 (1973).

5. S. Barone, *Appl. Opt.* 6, 861 (1967).

6. L. Bergstein, *Appl. Opt.* 7, 495 (1968).

7. W. Streifer, *IEEE* QE-4, 229 (1968).

8. A. G. Fox and T. Li, (a) *Proc. IEEE* S-1, 80 (1963);
    (b) *Quantum Electronics III*, New York, p. 1263,
    Columbia University Press (1964).

9. R. Sanderson and H. Streiger, (a) *Appl. Opt.* 8, 131
    (1969); (b) *Appl. Opt.* 8, 2129 (1969).

10. H. Kogelnik and T. Li, *Appl. Opt.* 5, 1550 (1966).

11. W. E. Lamb, Jr., *Phys. Rev.* 134, A1429 (1964).

12. See, for example, B. Rossi, *Optics*, p. 84, Addison
    Wesley, Reading, Mass. (1957).

13. I. Gradshteyn and I. Ryzhik, *Table of Integrals,
    Series, and Products*, Academic Press, New York, N.Y.
    (1965).

14. A. Messiah, *Quantum Mechanics*, Wiley (1966).

15. M. Abramowitz and I. A. Stegun, *Handbook of Mathematical Functions*, Dover (1965).

16. Yu. A. Anan'ev, *Sov. J. Quant. Elect.* 1, 565 (May/June 1972).

17. Yu. A. Anan'ev and V. E. Sherstobitov, *Sov. J. Quant. Elect.* 1, 263 (November/December 1971).

18. H. Zucker, *Bell Systems Tech. J.* 49, 2349-2376 (1970).

19. M. Lax, W. H. Louisell, C. Greninger, and W. B. McKnight, (Abstract H.2 only), *IEEE J. Quant. Elect.* QE-8, 554 (1973).

20. A. N. Chester, *Appl. Opt.* 11, 2584 (1972).

21. G. L. McAllister, D. K. Rice, and W. H. Steier, *J. Opt. Soc. Am.* 63, 502 (1973).

22. H. Shih, M. O. Scully, and P. V. Avizonis (to be published).

AMPLIFIER THEORY

F. A. Hopf

3.1. INTRODUCTION

Theories of laser amplifiers have, at least in simplified cases, been around for as long as laser theories.
The former have, however, received much less vigorous
treatment due to several factors. First, the experiments
tend to be very messy. Secondly, the amplifier theories
are usually not soluble analytically, and finally, until
very recently there have not been any interesting measurements of kinetic atomic times that are uniquely suited to
amplifiers. This latter aspect is perhaps the most critical, since it has been applications to atomic physics and
engineering that have spurred the large scale detailed work
in laser theory.

Amplifier theories, then, are to be viewed as being
crude on the scale of laser theories, and are intended primarily to provide qualitative statements of amplifier
behavior. Quantitative results can be obtained, but almost
invariably at the expense of numerical calculations which

77

can be either straightforward or extremely long and tedious.
The expense can be justified in applications, for example,
to controlled thermonuclear fusion (see Chapters 7-9),
where the pulse shape and size is critical to the fusion
"burn."

We begin by considering, in outline form, the constituent parts of an amplifier calculation. These can be
divided into three areas: the laser medium, the mode of
operation of the amplifier, and the nature of the input
field. Specifically the *laser medium* can have one or more
of the following:

   a.   two levels
   b.   degenerate multiple levels
   c.   homogeneous broadening
   d.   inhomogeneous broadening
   e.   adjacent levels (rotational sublevels)
   f.   losses
   g.   Kerr activity
   h.   spatial inhomogeneity.

The *mode of operation* can involve:

   a.   single pass
   b.   multiple passes
   c.   pumping prior to interaction
   d.   CW pumping
   e.   amplification on single line
   f.   amplification on many lines.

The *input field* can be:

   a.   pulsed with or without phase modulation and noise
   b.   CW with or without modulation and noise.

Clearly it is not possible to consider all of the
allowed combinations of possibilities that are included in
this outline. Fortunately, it is not necessary to do so
since laser systems of interest limit our concern to just a
few combinations. We concentrate on these significant

combinations and see that there are many areas in which
knowledge derived from one system can be applied directly
to another. In order to get the maximum mileage out of
these interrelationships, we consider the most difficult
problems first, and then specialize to the simpler ones.
For that reason, we treat primarily pulsed amplifiers,
since many aspects of CW operation can be understood fairly
easily with a knowledge of pulse operation. The only ex-
ception is our discussion of amplified spontaneous emission
in Sec. 3-4. In the remainder of this section, we summarize other sections and give the overall assumptions of the
theories we treat. In Sec. 3-2, we give the basic theory
of pulse amplification by two-level systems allowing for
both inhomogeneous and homogeneous broadening. Section 3-3
applies the theory of Sec. 3-2 to operation of amplifiers
with media like Nd^{+++}:Glass and ruby. In Sec. 3-4 we consider CW amplifiers and noise amplifiers ("superflourescent
lasers"). Section 3-5 treats molecular and chemical amplifiers with particular attention to CO_2, HF and CO systems.
Section 3-6 correlates references on the material of this
chapter. Various appendices elaborate on the material; in
particular, Appendix A relates amplifier theory to the
classical theory of absorption, and provides a notation
glossary.

There are various aspects of the amplifier model that
are common throughout this set of lectures. First, we pre-
tend that the wave is plane parallel light, i.e., we
neglect all variations transverse to the direction of propagation. The electric field is then describable as

$$E(t,z) = \frac{1}{2} E(t,z) \exp[i(kz-\nu t)] + \text{c.c.}, \tag{1}$$

where $E(t,z)$ is a complex envelope which varies little in an optical period and wavelength.

Although this model represents a set of measure zero with respect to real-world problems, the transverse behavior is potentially so complicated that no general discussion is feasible unless this model is used. The polarization in the medium is then written as

$$P(t,z) = \frac{1}{2} P(t,z) \exp[i(kz - \nu t)] + \text{c.c.}, \tag{2}$$

where $P(t,z)$ is a complex polarization envelope. This polarization is typically due to many different sources. We do not formally show how contributions other than those from the amplifying species itself come into the problem. They are introduced on an *ad hoc* basis when needed.

Throughout this discussion the field and polarization are taken to be quantities that vary little on the time and length scales given by $1/\nu$ and $1/k$. Formally, this means that if

$$E(t,z) = |E(t,z)| \exp[i\phi(t,z)], \tag{3}$$

then

$$\frac{\partial |E(t,z)|}{\partial z} \ll k|E(t,z)|; \qquad \frac{\partial |E(t,z)|}{\partial t} \ll \nu|E(t,z)|;$$

$$\frac{\partial \phi}{\partial z} \ll k; \qquad \frac{\partial \phi}{\partial t} \ll \nu. \tag{4}$$

This approximation is equivalent to saying that the bandwidth of the field is much smaller than its frequency, and
that the field does not grow or decay much in traveling a
wavelength.

The wave equation for a plane-wave configuration is
(see Sec. 3-6 for background references)

$$-\nabla^2 E + \frac{1}{c^2} \frac{\partial^2}{\partial t^2} E = \mu_o \frac{\partial^2}{\partial t^2} P. \qquad (5)$$

With the approximations of (4) and some care (see Appendix
A), we find

$$\frac{\partial E}{\partial z} + \frac{1}{c} \frac{\partial E}{\partial t} = -i \frac{\nu}{2E_o c} P - \kappa E. \qquad (6)$$

The loss term $-\kappa E$ has been included here on an *ad hoc* basis.
It is usually introduced by considering equally *ad hoc*
terms representing fictitious ohmic currents.

This is the "reduced wave equation" that is common to
our lectures. The only modifications occur in the value
and form of the complex polarizations. We usually calculate the polarization by means of a generalized susceptibility. We note that[1]

$$\tilde{P}(\omega,z) = \tilde{\chi}(\omega,z)\tilde{E}(\omega,z), \qquad (7)$$

where the tilded symbol indicates Fourier transforms. This
immediately gives

$$P(t,z) \;=\; \int_{-\infty}^{t} dt'\chi(t-t',z)E(t',z).\eqno(8)$$

In the more general problem, the susceptibility is time dependent, for which the polarization is given by

$$P(t,z) \;=\; \int_{-\infty}^{t} dt'\chi(t-t',t',z)E(t',z).\eqno(9)$$

We cannot now Fourier transform back to get Eq. (7). However, it always is possible to get the time dependence of the susceptibility through some kind of differential equation. We do not use the susceptibility in precisely this form, but try to normalize it allowing the length scale to be written explicitly in terms of a gain coefficient.

3.2. BASIC THEORY OF PULSE AMPLIFICATION BY TWO-LEVEL SYSTEMS

In this section, we start from the phenomenological Bloch equations and develop the equations and techniques of solution of the simplest pulsed cases (which are frequently the most difficult to solve). Background material is included in Appendix A and in Ref. 2. The Bloch equations are equivalent to the basic equations of the quantum-mechanical two-level atom, provided the upper and lower level decay times are the same, or else that they are sufficiently long not to matter. The latter condition is taken to be true for most of our work. We then write the equation of motion for the probability difference $W(\omega,t,z)$ as

$$\frac{\partial W}{\partial t} = -\frac{\wp}{2\hbar} P(\omega,t,z)E^*(t,z) + c.c., \tag{10}$$

and that for the complex polarization as

$$P(\omega,t,z) = -P(\omega,t,z)/T_2 - i(\omega-\nu)P + \frac{\wp E}{\hbar} W. \tag{11}$$

Here, $P(\omega,t,z)$ is the polarization contribution from an atom whose natural frequency is ω. Note that through local irregularities in a solid state matrix or through Doppler shifting in a gas, not all atoms have the same frequency. This process is called *Inhomogeneous Broadening*, or IB for short. It comes into the problem via a distribution function $\sigma(\omega)$ which describes the probability of finding an atom with a resonant frequency ω. The dipole decay time T_2 leads to a *Homogeneous Broadening* (HB). The macroscopic polarization is then

$$P(t,z) = \int d\omega \alpha(\omega) P(\omega,t,z). \tag{12}$$

For our present purposes, it is sufficient to take the distribution $\sigma(\omega)$ to be Gaussian with a center of symmetry at ω_o. In that case, we can *normalize* the problem by choosing a carrier frequency

$$\nu = \omega_o, \tag{13}$$

and refer all frequencies to ν. Any nonresonant aspects of the problem are then included in the phase ϕ of Eq. (3). The inhomogeneous distribution is best characterized by the Fourier transform $D(T)$ of the inhomogeneous frequency distribution

$$D(T) = \frac{1}{2\pi\sigma(\omega_o)} \int d\omega \sigma(\omega) \exp[-i(\omega-\omega_o)T]$$

$$= \frac{1}{\sqrt{\pi}T_2^*} \exp[-T^2/T_2^{*2}] \tag{14}$$

$$\sigma(\omega) = \frac{T_2^*}{2\sqrt{\pi}} \exp[-(\omega-\omega_o)^2 T_2^{*2}/4]. \tag{15}$$

In this context, the meaning of susceptibility [i.e., $\chi(\omega) \sim \sigma(\omega)$] is redefined in terms of the equivalent meaning of a decay, in time, of a phased array of dipoles. The generalized nonlinear susceptibility is found by rewriting the polarization as

$$P(\omega,t,z) = \frac{\wp}{\hbar} \int_{-\infty}^{t} dt' E(t',z) \exp[-(t-t')/T_2]$$

$$\times \exp[-i(\omega-\omega_o)(t-t')]W(\omega,t',z). \tag{16}$$

When this is integrated over frequencies to give the macroscopic polarization, the underlined quantity represents a
Fourier transform over the frequency ω that leads to the
susceptibility operator. Note that $D(T)$ is normalized to
unity, and we make the normalization for χ work the same
way. This then gives

$$\frac{\partial E}{\partial z} + \frac{1}{c}\frac{\partial E}{\partial t} = \alpha \int_{-\infty}^{t} dt' \underline{\chi(t-t',t',z)}$$

$$\times \ \underline{\exp[-(t-t')/T_2]E(t',z)}, \tag{17}$$

where α is the gain coefficient in the limit $T_2 \to \infty$. Note
that the specific formula for α depends upon the context.
Here it is

$$\alpha = \wp^2 N \nu \pi \sigma(\omega_o)/2c\varepsilon_o \hbar.$$

The susceptibility [underlined in Eq. (16)]
is broken into two parts. The inhomogeneous part is
represented by χ and the homogeneous part is given by the
exponential which we discuss later. The IB part of the
susceptibility is defined as

$$\chi(T,t,z) \equiv \frac{1}{2\pi\sigma(\omega_o)} \int d\omega \sigma(\omega) W(\omega,t,z) \exp[-i(\omega-\omega_o)T], \tag{18}$$

and has the normalization property

$$\int dT \chi(T,t,z) \;=\; W(\omega_o,t,z). \tag{19}$$

At t_o = time just before the pulse arrives, $W(\omega,t_o,z)$ = +1, so that

$$\chi(T,t_o,z) \;=\; D(T).$$

Similarly, if the electric field is very small, then $\dot{W}$ = 0 and the susceptibility retains the value $D(T)$ throughout the interaction. If one ignores T_2 by setting $T_2 \to \infty$, and takes the pulse to be resonant with a width $\hat{t}$ long compared to T_2^*, then $\chi(T,t,z) = D(T)$ acts like a delta function in (17). One gets

$$\frac{\partial E}{\partial z} + \frac{1}{c}\frac{\partial E}{\partial t} \;=\; \frac{\alpha}{2}\,E(t,z). \tag{20}$$

Multiplying both sides by $(\wp^2/\hbar^2)E^*$, we get an expression for I which is proportional to the power

$$\frac{\partial I(t,z)}{\partial z} + \frac{1}{c}\frac{\partial I(t,z)}{\partial t} \;=\; \alpha I; \qquad I \;=\; \left|\wp\frac{E}{\hbar}\right|^2. \tag{21}$$

One can integrate this in time to get the energy $[T(z)]$ position rate of change:

$$\frac{dT}{dz} \;=\; \alpha T,$$

where the energy $T(z)$ is defined to be

$$T \equiv \int_{-\infty}^{\infty} dt' I(t',z) . \tag{22}$$

The energy and power here are defined in "atomic" units, which conveniently describe the interaction of light and matter. Since they involve the dipole matrix element $\wp$, there is no unique general relationship between these units and MKS. Instead, they vary from one pair of levels to another. Equations (20)-(22) describe the small signal (Beer's law--see Ref. 2) for the amplifier. Then α is the gain coefficient which is given by

$$\alpha = \frac{\wp^2 \nu N \pi \sigma (\omega_o)}{\hbar c \varepsilon_o} . \tag{23}$$

The nonlinear behavior is determined by an equation of motion for $\chi(T,t,z)$ which is found in a straightforward way by substituting $P(\omega,t,z)$ [Eq. (16)] into Eq. (10) and using the definition (18) for χ. Thus,

$$\frac{\partial \chi(T,t,z)}{\partial t} = -\frac{\wp^2}{2\hbar^2} \int_{-\infty}^{t} dt' \exp[-(t-t')/T_2] [E(t,z)E^*(t',z)$$

$$\times \chi^*(T-t+t',t',z) + E^*(t,z)E(t',z)\chi(T+t-t',t',z)] . \tag{24}$$

In general, this somewhat formidable integro-differential equation must be solved numerically.

Appendix B derives one important relationship that represents the general conservation of energy law, namely,

$$\frac{\partial I}{\partial z} + \frac{1}{c}\frac{\partial I}{\partial t} = -\alpha \frac{\hbar^2}{\wp^2}\frac{\partial \chi(0,t,z)}{\partial t} . \tag{25}$$

This is precisely what one would expect since $\chi(0,t,z)$ is,
by definition, simply the integral over the inhomogeneous
line of the population of the levels. In MKS units, this
says that every time an atom makes a transition down (or
up), a "photon" is added (removed) from the field.

These equations, as noted previously, contain the
Homogeneous Broadening or HB as well as the IB part. The
decay time T_2 (i.e., the HB) represents phase destroying
collisions that disrupt the coherence between the atom and
field. In our approximation, they affect all atoms equally,
hence the term homogeneous. These equations contain both
parts, which we refer to as *Mixed Broadening* (MB) which is
exclusively the province of numerical calculations and is
not extensively discussed in this section. We have reason
later on to deal with an unbroadened or *Power Broadened*
(PB) medium which represents the situation in which neither
T_2 nor T_2^* processes play a role.

Homogeneously Broadened Amplifier

In the case of pure HB, the amplifier equations are
structured somewhat differently. We have $\sigma(\omega) = \delta(\omega-\omega_o)$
which says that $D(T)$ and $\chi(T,t,z)$ are independent of T.
This suggests replacing these with a quantity which is
dependent on t and z and measures the inversion. The

candidate in this case is obvious, namely the quantity
$W(\omega_0,t,z) = n(t,z)$ which is the inversion of the single
natural frequency of the homogeneous line. The substitution $\chi(T,t,z) = n(t,z)D(T)$ preserves the normalization, and
gives (noting $D(T) = $ constant)

$$\frac{\partial E}{\partial z} + \frac{1}{c}\frac{\partial E}{\partial t} = \alpha' \int_{-\infty}^{t} dt' \underline{\exp[-(t-t')/T_2]n(t',z)E(t',z)},$$
(26)

where

$$\alpha' = \frac{\wp^2 n\nu}{2\hbar c\varepsilon_0}.$$
(27)

Again, we have underlined the generalized nonlinear
susceptibility as it appears in this equation. The susceptibility is defined by our knowledge of the behavior of the
inversion which is given by the equation

$$\dot{n}(t,z) = -\frac{\wp^2}{2\hbar^2} \int_{-\infty}^{t} dt' [E(t,z)E^*(t',z) + \text{c.c.}]$$

$$\times\ n(t',z)\exp[-(t-t')/T_2].$$
(28)

This equation, even though it is much simpler than
before, still is not soluble except by numerical techniques.
If, in this case, we perform the same small-signal calculation as for Eqs. (20)-(22), take T_2 to be much shorter than
the pulse width and let $n = 1 = $ constant, we find that we

get the same Beer's Law relationships [(20)-(22)] except
that the gain coefficient

$$\alpha = 2\alpha' T_2, \tag{29}$$

where α' is given by (23).

Note that, in the case of MB, the gain is given by

$$\alpha = 2\alpha' \int_0^\infty dT \; \exp[-T/T_2]D(T). \tag{30}$$

This is the time-domain description of the plasma dispersion function, a quantity that represents the convolution
(in frequency) of the homogeneous- and inhomogeneous-line
functions.

In Sec. 3.3, we are concerned with the detailed solution of these coupled equations of motion. For the rest of
this section, we recast the equations into the time-
retarded frame and investigate simple but important
consequences.

The first transformation concerns the peculiar derivative that appears on the left-hand side of the reduced wave
equation (6) which we write here without the loss term as

$$\frac{\wp}{\hbar} \left(\frac{\partial}{\partial z} + \frac{1}{c} \frac{\partial}{\partial t} \right) E(t,z) = \alpha' P(t,z). \tag{31}$$

This is known as a convective derivative, and says that an
event that takes place at a space-time point (z,t) has an
effect at the point $(z + \Delta z, \; t + \Delta z/c)$. This derivative is

well-known in electrodynamics, and we do the same thing
here that is done there: namely use the retarded time μ

$$\mu = t - \frac{z}{c} .$$ (32)

With the substitution $t \rightarrow \mu$, Eq. (31) becomes

$$\frac{\wp}{\hbar} \frac{\partial}{\partial z} E(\mu,z) = \alpha' P(\mu,z) .$$ (33)

Note that if $\alpha' = 0$ (no atoms), the pulse does not
change. Hence, the retarded time is called the *Rest Frame
of the Pulse*. Note that for the equation of motion of the
medium, one just substitutes t for μ. This frame is the
most useful one for analytic work, and is the best frame
for computer solutions as well (see Appendix C).

In every problem in electrodynamics, there is an
advanced solution that is the same as the retarded one
except that time appears to flow backwards. Thus, for an
input pulse $E(\mu,0)$ that gives rise to a field $E(\mu,z)$ and
polarization $P(\mu,z)$ [and ultimately to an output pulse
$E(\mu,L)$], there is a solution in which μ is replaced every-
where by $(t + z/c)$. Note that the latter has a straightforward interpretation as an attenuator with an input
$E(t + L/c,L)$ and an output $E(t,0)$. This means that for
every amplifier, there corresponds an attenuator[10] (found by
replacing α or α' by $-\alpha$ or $-\alpha'$) which takes the output
pulse from the amplifier and generates the input.

It is frequently the case in short pulse problems that
one is interested in a particular kind of output pulse.

For example, one may want a zero-π pulse for low-loss propagation or a ramp pulse for optimum compression of a plasma
(see Chap. 9).   Instead of a "hunt and peck" technique of
trying many different inputs to find the output, one can
use the desired output and pass it through the equivalent
attenuator to find the input that one needs. This procedure cannot be applied with complete generality since it is
sometimes the case that a stable pulse in the amplifier
turns out to be unstable in the attenuator and vice versa.
This instability is not usually a problem in practical
cases, but is rather a property of more esoteric systems.

There are the usual transformations of the equations
of motion to dimensionless units which frequently provide
interesting results. The first transformation concerns
spatial nonuniformities in gain (we consider longitudinal
only, no transverse) that frequently occur in amplifiers.
This is described by an α or α' that is a function of z.
One can use the variable

$$\xi = \int_0^z dz' \alpha'(z')$$

to transform the equation.   One gets

$$\frac{\wp}{\hbar} \frac{\partial E(\mu,\xi)}{\partial \xi} = P(\mu,\xi). \tag{34}$$

This says that the field is a function of ξ (i.e., the
integrated gain) and is not affected by spatial inhomo-
geneities in the medium.

In the time-domain aspect of the pulse, it is possible to transform to dimensionless coordinates $\mu/T_2{}^*$ or μ/T_2 in the IB or HB amplifier. This means that all of the variables are relative to their respective time scales, and are not functions of the absolute value of the times. Thus, a solution for a dilute (Doppler broadened) gas with $T_2{}^* \sim 10$ nsec can be applied, for example, to Nd^{+++} glass, $T_2{}^* \sim .3$ psec provided no other effects come into play. (Unfortunately, there are other effects which will be discussed in Sec. 3.3 below.) There is, however, a large regime of interest within the limit of pressure broadened gases in which the time constants span the range 10 nsec $\geq T_2 \geq 0.1$ nsec. Within this range, it does seem possible to be able to scale the results as indicated by the substitution $\mu \rightarrow \mu/T_2$. Note that this same range covers the present limit of electronic diagnostics. Thus, one can perform experiments in a low pressure regime (~ 30 Torr) where diagnostics are available, and, with some confidence of success, scale the results to regimes (~ 1 atm) where diagnostics are difficult.

3.3. AMPLIFIER OPERATION

In this section, we discuss the results of simple two-level atom models of the sort for which the equations developed in the previous section are suitable. In particular, the HB medium is a suitable model for ruby (at room temperature), and the IB medium is suitable for Nd^{+++} glass. We discuss the HB case first because it is easier.

The Homogeneously Broadened Amplifier (Ruby)

The HB amplifier is described by the equations of motion (26) and (28). In the "rest frame" coordinates z and μ, these are written as

$$\frac{\partial E(\mu,z)}{\partial z} = \alpha' \int_{-\infty}^{\mu} d\mu' e^{-(\mu-\mu')/T_2} E(\mu',z)n(\mu',z) \quad (35)$$

$$\frac{\partial n}{\partial \mu} = -\frac{\wp^2}{2\hbar^2} \int_{-\infty}^{\mu} d\mu'[E(\mu,z)E^*(\mu',z) + c.c.]$$

$$\times \exp[-(\mu-\mu')/T_2]n(\mu',z). \quad (36)$$

The model admits to the only limit in which the transient propagation problem is analytically soluble. This limit occurs when the pulse width $\hat{t}$ is much longer than T_2 (also the phase varies slowly compared to T_2). In that case, Eq. (36) becomes

$$\frac{\partial n}{\partial \mu} = -T_2 In, \quad (37)$$

where $I = (\wp E/h)^2$. Similarly, the equation of motion for the optical field intensity becomes

$$\frac{\partial I}{\partial z} = \alpha nI. \quad (38)$$

We refer to these as "rate equations" since they have
the typical form of chemical kinetic equations or radioac-
tive decay equations. They are the simplest possible equations that one can write down for the amplifier. Although
there isn't a wide class of problems for which they are
suited, slightly generalized versions are most useful for
the molecular amplifier discussed in Sec. 5.

These equations are solved by first writing the formal
solution of Eq. (37)

$$n(\mu,z) = \exp\left[-T_2 \int_0^\mu d\mu' I(\mu',z)\right]. \tag{39}$$

Here, we have defined $\mu = 0$ as a time just before the pulse
arrives, and the initial condition for the medium is then
$n(0,z) = 1$. This equation tells us one important fact,
namely that n can never be negative. This says that in
this limit it is impossible to extract more than half of
the stored energy. This can be seen by letting N_a be the
number of atoms in the upper state initially and letting
the lower state be unpopulated. Then, the best one can do
in extracting energy is to let the upper and lower states
have equal populations (this is what is meant by zero inversion). The extracted energy is given by the number of
atoms that make the transition, which is given by the number that wind up in the lower state, and this is $N_a/2$.
Thus, the extracted energy is $(N_a/2)\hbar\nu$. Substituting
Eq. (39) into Eq. (38) and integrating in time to get the
total energy, one finds

$$dT/dz = 2\alpha'[1 - \exp(-T_2 T)]. \tag{40}$$

This equation says that the output energy is a function only of the input energy. This is a property that is unique to this model; in all other cases, the output energy is very hard to specify in such a general way. Equation (40) can be solved in closed form to give

$$T(L) = \frac{1}{T_2} \text{Log}_e \{1 + (\exp[T_2 T(0)] - 1)e^{\alpha L}\}, \qquad (41)$$

where $\alpha = 2\alpha' T_2$ is the gain coefficient for small signal. There are two descriptive quantities that are useful in describing the amplifier: (1) the enhancement

$$E = T(L)/T(0) \qquad (42)$$

which measures the growth in the pulse, and (2) the efficiency

$$\eta = [T(L) - T(0)]/\text{Stored Energy}. \qquad (43)$$

It is straightforward (but algebraically nontrivial) to show that the maximum rate of growth occurs when the input signal is very small, and the pulse obeys Beer's Law (see Sec. 3.2). The maximum efficiency occurs in the other limit, namely when $T(0)$ is very large. This is referred to as the limit of total saturation. Using the fact that only half of the stored energy can be extracted in this limit, we can find the stored energy. From Eq. (40) we see that

$$T(L) - T(0) = \frac{\alpha L}{T_2} . \qquad (44)$$

Further using the relationship (29) between α and α', we
see that the total stored energy per unit volume (unit
volume and unit length are the same here) is $4\alpha'$, and
therefore that the maximum that can be extracted is $2\alpha'$.

The pulse wave-forms can also be treated in closed
form in this model. For the input wave-form $I(\mu,0)$, the
output is given by

$$I(\mu,L) = \frac{I(\mu,0)e^{\alpha L}\exp\left[T_2\int_0^\mu d\mu' I(0,\mu')\right]}{1 + e^{\alpha L}\left\{\exp\left[T_2\int_0^\mu d\mu' I(0,\mu')\right] - 1\right\}} . \qquad (45)$$

In Figs. 1a and 1b, we show the outputs for various
lengths of amplifiers resulting from input pulses which are
Gaussian and hyperbolic secant respectively. One can see
that there are several changes that may occur. The pulse
widths can either increase or decrease. The peak power
always increases, but may not increase much, and the location of the peak of the pulse shifts forward, giving an
apparent pulse velocity greater than the velocity of light.
Generally speaking, these phenomena tend to group into two
characteristic combinations. If the rise time of the pulse
is slow, as in the use of the hyperbolic secant, one has
large peak shifts with little or no narrowing nor any
particular increase in peak power. If the rise time is
fast, then the situation reverses, with increasing peak
power, some narrowing and little peak motion.

In the latter case, the pulse slowly narrows until the
condition $\hat{t} \ll T_2$ is no longer satisfied. At that point,

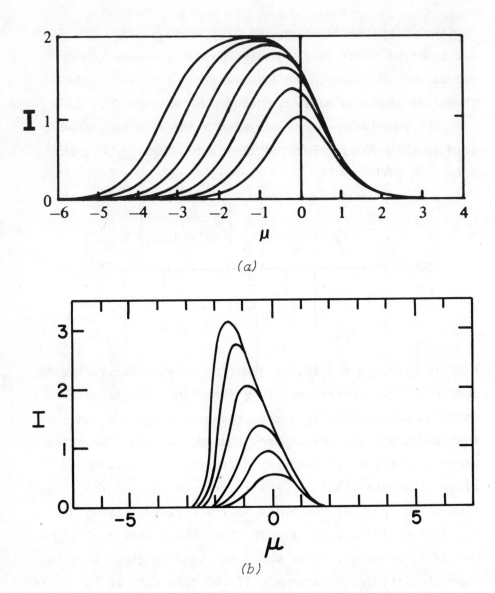

Fig. 1.   (a) Evolution of a hyperbolic secant pulse as
          given by Eq. (45) in an amplifying medium. The
          distances z are 0, 1/α, 2/α, ... 6/α in order of
          increasing intensity. From Ref. 2, Chap. 13; see
          Prob. 13-9 of that text for specific formula.
          (b) Same as 1(a), but for Gaussian Input.

atomic coherence becomes important. By this we mean that the atoms contain in their response a specific memory of the phase of the electromagnetic wave at earlier times. This considerably complicates the problem and makes it, in so far as detailed calculations are concerned, almost exclusively the province of numerical calculations. There are a few analytic results which are applicable in limiting cases. This involves considering the opposite extreme $\hat{t} << T_2$ which is the Power (or unbroadened) Medium (PB) limit.

In this limit, T_2 disappears from the equations (35) and (36) yielding the equation of motion

$$\frac{\partial n}{\partial \mu} = -\frac{\wp^2}{2\hbar^2} \int_{-\infty}^{\mu} d\mu' [E(\mu,z)E^*(\mu',z) + \text{c.c.}]n(\mu',z). \quad (46)$$

This equation is soluble in closed form for simple pulse envelopes. In general, one has the envelope

$$E(\mu,z) = |E(\mu,z)|e^{i\phi(\mu,z)}. \quad (47)$$

The simplification involves setting $\phi(\mu,z) = 0°$ or $180°$. This condition is called the *Zero* (sic) *Phase Approximation* and converts the pulse envelope into a real number. Rather than trying to hang onto phase flips explicitly, it is much better to represent them by noting that $e^{i\pi} = -1$, and thus, one can simply let $E(\mu,z)$ become negative. Under these circumstances, the complex conjugates in Eq. (46) go away and one finds that

$$n(\mu,z) \;=\; \cos\left\{\int_{-\infty}^{\mu} d\mu' \; \frac{\wp E(\mu',z)}{\hbar}\right\}. \tag{48}$$

Similarly, one gets an equation of motion for the field

$$\frac{\wp}{\hbar}\frac{\partial E}{\partial z} \;=\; \alpha' \sin\left\{\int_{-\infty}^{\mu} d\mu' \; \frac{\wp E(\mu',z)}{\hbar}\right\}. \tag{49}$$

Note from Eq. (48) that there is no longer a constraint on the inversion which can now become negative and hence, more energy can be extracted than in the rate equation approximation. This is shown by the formula for the development of the energy

$$\frac{dT}{dz} \;=\; 2\alpha'(1 - \cos\theta), \tag{50}$$

where

$$\theta \;=\; \int_{-\infty}^{\infty} d\mu \; \frac{\wp E(\mu,z)}{\hbar} \tag{51}$$

is the *area* of the pulse. If the area of the pulse is π, then one can extract $4\alpha'$ from the medium (i.e., all the available energy). This equation has a solution of the form $E(\mu z)$[13] (NOTE: this is a product, the comma is not missing) with the property $\theta = \pi$. This solution has the property that the time scale of the pulse decreases in length as $1/z$ and the peak power increases as z^2. This property

is the principal characteristic of *Superradiance* and the PB
medium bears a close relationship to Dicke's original
model.[3]   Note that the time structure of the pulse narrows
indefinitely. This implies a continued increase in the
spectral width of the pulse which seems peculiar in view of
the small bandwidth of the amplifier. This is the origin
of the use of Power *Broadening* of the Medium as the source
of the large pulse spectrum. The pulse itself is shown in
Fig. 2 at some arbitrary point (the solution, by definition,
has a constant shape).   Note the strong ringing on the
trailing edge. This ringing prevents describing the pulse
evolution simply as a constant narrowing. The individual
spikes in the pulse contain only small portions of the
overall energy.

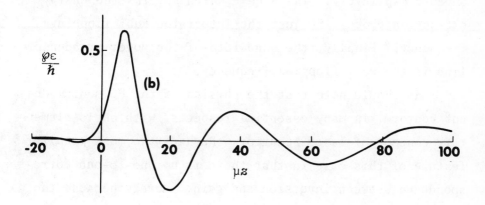

Fig. 2. Output waveform in power broadened medium.

The physics of the coherent interaction is contained
in the fact that the medium responds to the integral over
the field amplitude. Let us consider a special case of a

step function ($E = 0$ for $\mu \le 0$; $E = E_O$, $\mu \ge 0$) input incident on a rarified gas. In that case, Eq. (49) can be
solved by a Taylor's expansion to first order and the time
integral can be done easily. One finds

$$\frac{\wp E(\mu,L)}{\hbar} = \frac{\wp E_O}{\hbar} + \alpha' L \sin\left[\frac{\wp E_O}{\hbar}\mu\right]. \tag{52}$$

The output is then a constant field with a ripple on the
surface. This ripple is called an *Optical Nutation*. The
oscillation in polarization (and population) that causes
the ripple is called the *Rabi Flopping Effect* and the
quantity $\wp E_O/\hbar$ is called the *Rabi Flopping Frequency*. This
is an extremely important quantity in all aspects of amplifier operation, and that is the reason we have been careful
to always write the equations so that the factor $\wp/\hbar$
appears explicitly. The area θ which governs the energy
extraction process is just the integrated Rabi flopping
frequency. Finally, the bandwidth of the power broadened
line is the Rabi flopping frequency.

One should note that the physics of the PB medium does
not conform, in many essential respects, with one's elementary concept of laser behavior. Perhaps the most peculiar
feature of this case is that there is no one-to-one corre-
spondence between inversion and gain. Merely because the
inversion is negative at some instant in time (i.e., more
atoms in lower than upper state), it does not follow that
the pulse is losing energy to the atoms (nor does it follow
that positive inversions imply instantaneous gain).
Clearly any attempt to understand the effects of atomic
coherence demands an abandonment of preconceived notions.

To summarize, the HB amplifier can be discussed in two regimes. In the long pulse regime, rate equations can be used, yielding a well-behaved energy function (i.e., enhancements and efficiencies are predictable), but it is not straightforward to make short widths and high peak powers. In the limit of extremely short pulses, one sees a picture of increased efficiency, narrowing of the time scale of the pulse, and large increases in power. The intermediate regime (widths $\sim T_2$) has received considerable detailed study, all numerical, none of which has appeared in the literature. In this third case, there is a straightforward blend of the two limits. Powers always increase, narrowing always occurs (but not as much as in the PB limit). The trailing edge ripples are greatly suppressed. The energy is not well behaved (i.e., it is a function of all pulse parameters), and the potential efficiency lies between the two limits.

Inhomogeneously Broadened Amplifiers (Nd^{+++} Glass)

The theoretical discussion of the IB amplifiers represents the worst possible combination of the difficulties encountered in the HB effect. First, there is the inhomogeneous broadening time constant T_2^* so that the PB limit is not valid; on the other hand, atomic coherence plays an important role so there is no long pulse in which rate equations apply. There are two rays of sunshine in all of this. If one works with the zero phase assumption, the pulse area (51) obeys the *McCall-Hahn Area Theorem*[5]

$$(d\theta/dz) = (\alpha/2)\sin\theta. \qquad (53)$$

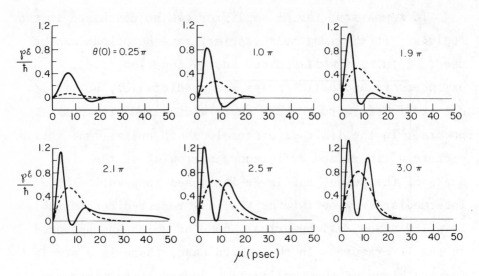

Fig. 3. *Output pulses (solid line) that result from input
pulses (broken line) with different values of
input area. The input areas are given in the
labels of the figures. The corresponding values
of the input integrated intensity* $\tau(0)$ *are (a)*
0.089 psec^{-1}, *(b)* 0.62 psec^{-1}, *(c)* 2.24 psec^{-1},
(d) 2.74 psec^{-1}, *(e)* 3.88 psec^{-1}, *and (f)*
5.60 psec^{-1}.

One can also derive a modified version of Eq. (52)
which shows that there is an optical nutation effect in
this case. Thus, in view of the close resemblance of the
physics in each case to the physics of the mixed broadening,
one might expect that there is a similarity in the results.
In Fig. 3, we show typical outputs for this case which
point out both similarities and differences. First, there
is considerable narrowing in this case, and the subsequent
ringing is usually, but not always, sufficiently small so
that the notion of pulse width is well defined. There is
also a noticeable increase in peak power. In Fig. 4, the
energy is shown as a function of distance down the rod. We

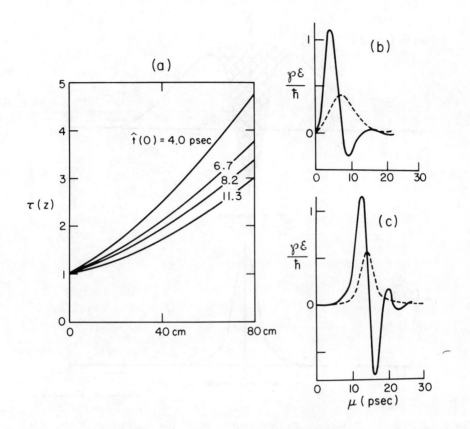

Fig. 4. *There are four pulse configurations considered in this figure. They have a fixed input integrated intensity $\tau(0)$, with the varied input parameters given as (i) $\hat{t}(0)$ = 11.3 psec, $\theta(0)$ = 3.99; (ii) $\hat{t}(0)$ = 8.2 psec, $\theta(0)$ = 3.44; (iii) $\hat{t}(0)$ = 6.7 psec, $\theta(0)$ = 3.13; and (iv) $\hat{t}(0)$ = 4.0 psec, $\theta(0)$ = 2.72. The shapes of the first three input pulse shapes are similar to those in Fig. 3 with exponents of 1, 2, and 3, respectively. Case (iv) is a hyperbolic secant. (a) depicts the value of $\tau(z)$ versus z for the four pulses; (b) is the output pulse (solid line) for the case (ii) (broken line); and (c) is the same as (b) for case (iv).*

see what is meant by the development of the energy not being well defined. In each case, the input energy is the same, but there is considerable variation in output.

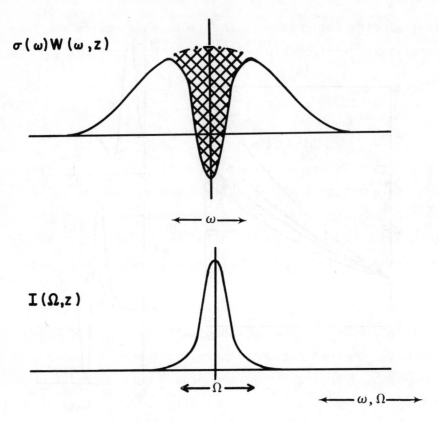

Fig. 5.   *Hole Burning Schematic: The original line (_._.)*
          is pushed down leaving a hole (cross-hatched) in
          the line. The width of the hole is approximately
          the spectral width of the pulse.

In this case, it is fairly straightforward to see why
this variation occurs. In the IB medium, the pulse affects
primarily atoms which are resonant within the bandwidth of
the pulse. This results in a phenomenon called *hole*
burning, which is shown in Fig. 5. There is a large piece
of the initial line that is eaten away by the pulse. The
magnitude of this hole can be determined by noting that its
width is given by $1/\hat{t}$ and its depth by $1 - \cos\theta$. Conservation of energy says that the change in energy is just the

integral over the change in the line, which gives an
approximate relationship

$$\frac{dT}{dz} \approx \frac{2\alpha}{\hat{t}}(1 - \cos\theta)C, \tag{54}$$

where C is a factor of the order unity given by the dimensionless quantity $T\hat{t}/\theta^2$ which is dependent on the pulse
shape. Thus, the efficiency is dependent on the pulse
width and area, so it is not at all surprising that merely
specifying the input energy is insufficient to determine
the output.

There are many other aspects to transient behavior in
the IB amplifier of considerable interest and importance
that have not been discussed here. However, from the
standpoint of applications, the glass laser is beset by a
host of other difficulties whose effects are not yet completely understood. These produce phase fluctuations whose
role is discussed in Sec. 4.

In summary, the development of nonphase modulated
pulses can be divided into two regimes in which atomic
coherence does and does not play a role. In the absence of
atomic coherence, there is, at best, a rather poor capability for pulse narrowing and peak power growth. In some
instances, these may not occur to any extent at all. In
the limit where atomic coherence is important, there
generally is a great deal of narrowing and increasing peak
power, but the narrowing may have to be viewed with skepti-
cism in some cases. Generally speaking, the best pulse
intensification occurs in the IB medium which suggests that

glass lasers might be ideal for this application. In the
remainder of this section, we see that this isn't so.

Frequency Modulation in Pulse Propagation
A Critique of Nd^{+++} Glass

So far we have concentrated on the propagation of
pulses in the absence of phase modulation. The moment that
one admits to the possibility of nonzero time varying
phases, there arises a whole host of problems involving
such elementary questions as the meaning of amplitude and
frequency modulation on a pulse. In this chapter, there is
not sufficient time to ponder these in detail. Consequently we discuss with as little algebra as possible, just
one simple case, namely the Gaussian pulse with a linear
frequency sweep.

Ignoring, for the moment, the role of the amplifying
medium in a solid state laser, we recognize that the host
medium has an index of refraction that is a function of
both frequency and field amplitude. Thus, one can write a
Taylor's expansion of the host index

$$n = n_0 + n_1(\omega-\omega_o) + n_2(\omega-\omega_o)^2 + \ldots + n_k|E|^2 + \ldots .$$

$$(55)$$

These terms give rise to the phase velocity (n_0), group
velocity [$n_1(\omega-\omega_o)$], dispersive effects [$n_2(\omega-\omega_o)$], and
self-phase modulation ($n_k|E|^2$) (this last term also gives
rise to a power dependent group velocity). The key terms
for our purposes are the last two. The dispersive term has
the effect of causing a pulse which has no phase modulation

initially to acquire modulation as it propagates through
the medium.[4] It does this without changing the power spectrum $I(\Omega,z)$ defined by

$$I(\Omega,z) \;=\; |\int \frac{\wp}{\hbar} E(t,z)e^{-i\Omega t}dt|^2 . \tag{56}$$

This means that the amplitude modulation of the pulse is
converted into frequency modulation. For a simple waveform,
the pulse must therefore stretch out. In the case of a
Gaussian, the phase is very simple, and takes the form

$$\frac{d\phi}{dz} \;=\; \sqrt{1 - \gamma^2} \;(\mu-\mu_o), \tag{57}$$

where μ_o is the center of the pulse and the compression
factor

$$\gamma \;=\; \sqrt{1 + \frac{Dz}{\hat{t}_m^{\,2}}} . \tag{58}$$

Here D is a coefficient related to n_2, and $\hat{t}_m$ is the width
of the Gaussian when it still had zero phase. The derivative of the phase is the instantaneous frequency, and
Eq. (57) describes a linear frequency sweep or chirp. The
compression factor γ measures the ratio of the amplitude
and phase modulation in the pulse. Another meaning of γ is
the amount by which a pulse can be compressed using a
grating pair (see Treacy[6]).

The Kerr term (i.e., the power dependent index) causes
a frequency sweep of a somewhat different kind. For a

lossless Kerr effect, the equation of motion can be written

$$\frac{\partial E}{\partial z} = i\chi_K \frac{\wp^2}{\hbar^2} |E|^2 E ,$$
(59)

where χ_K is some appropriate coefficient. This has a solution

$$E(\mu,z) = E(\mu,0)\exp[i\chi_K zI(\mu,0)].$$
(60)

The frequency is the derivative in time of the term in the exponential which in turn, is just the derivative of the power. If the pulse rises and falls in a normal fashion, the frequency is an "S"-shaped curve, lying on its side. Note that the amplitude is not affected by this process, that is, a Kerr chirp develops with constant amplitude.

With the glass laser, there are two reasons why one expects very narrow pulses. First, it has a very wide (~100 Å) bandwidth, and secondly it is inhomogeneously broadened. However, short pulses run afoul of the two dispersive sources. The scaling law of host dispersion (i.e., the development of γ) indicates that short pulses disperse very rapidly. It turns out that pulses ~10^{-13} - 10^{-12} sec disperse over lengths of glass of the order of 10 to 100 cm. Similarly, very short pulses imply high powers which brings the Kerr effect into the pulse development in a major way.

It is not feasible at this time to attempt a general discussion of the simultaneous generation and amplification of chirped pulses. We note one example in Fig. 6 in which the pulse evolves in an IB amplifier with Kerr effect only. The lack of decrease in width and increase in peak power

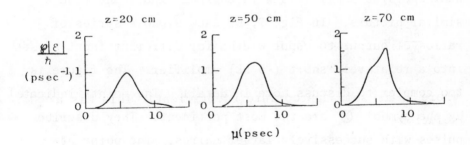

Fig. 6. *Gaussian pulse evolution in a Kerr host inhomogeneous amplifier.*

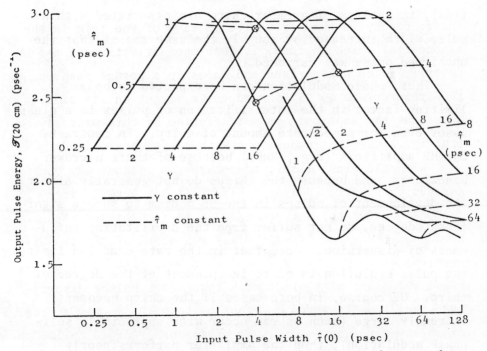

Fig. 7. *Normalized output pulse width versus input pulse width for various compression factors in a 20 cm inhomogeneous amplifier.*

are the most noticeable features from the standpoint of the present discussion. Instead of trying to solve the combined dispersive amplifier problem, we consider

nondispersive amplifiers with chirped inputs and find a
similar picture. In Fig. 7, we show a whole series of
ratios of output to input widths for different input pulses
into a relatively short (~5 DB) amplifier. The figure is
too complex to discuss here in detail. The points indicated
by the symbol ⊗ are the most pertinent. They describe
pulses with successively larger chirps. The point at
$\hat{t}(0) = 8$ is unchirped, and considering how short the amplifier is, has a non-negligible degree of narrowing. In contrast, the points of greater chirp are associated with a
pulse width increased by roughly the same amount that the
unchirped pulse was narrowed.

Thus, phase modulation can be expected to be a
limiting factor in the intensification of pulses in a glass
laser even for a moderate amount of chirp. In contrast,
the HB amplifiers (e.g., Ruby) because of their narrower
bandwidths, and because the chirps do not generally affect
the development of pulses in the HB medium to such a significant degree, do not suffer from the debilitating influences of dispersion. Note that in the rate equation limit,
the pulse evolution is quite independent of the degree of
chirp. Of course, in both cases if the chirp becomes
extremely large (such as can occur with appreciable self-
phase modulation), then the amplifier performs poorly
independently of the type of medium.

3.4. CW AND NOISE AMPLIFIERS (NITROGEN)

The CW amplifier is distinguished from the pulsed amplifier by virtue of a pump source which replenishes the atoms in the upper state that are lost either by natural decay or by the action of the optical field. We assume this pump is constant in time. Clearly, however, the present discussion can also be applied to time varying pumps provided the variation is slow compared to decay times, etc. The pump is introduced as an additional term in the right-hand side of the equations of motion of the form

$$\frac{\partial \chi(T,t,z)}{\partial t} = \Big(D(T) - \chi(T,t,z)\Big)/T_1 - \dots , \tag{61}$$

$$\frac{\partial n(t,z)}{\partial t} = \Big(1 - n(t,z)\Big)/T_1 - \dots , \tag{62}$$

for the IB and HB media respectively. The rest of the terms are the same as in (24) and (28), and the equations for the electromagnetic field are unchanged. Here, T_1 is the natural life-time of the upper and lower levels (taken to be the same). There is a particularly simple solution of these equations which describes the evolution of a mono-chromatic beam in an HB medium. This is a convenient place to start, and also provides a convenient point of contact with laser theory. The monochromatic solution says that the electric field amplitude is independent of time $[E(\mu,z) \rightarrow E(z)]$. Furthermore, for the amplitude to remain monochromatic, the population difference must be independent of time $[n(\mu,z) \rightarrow n(z)]$. We consider this second point in more detail later. All of the unknown quantities being independent of time, the various integrals can be done trivially. We find for the HB case that

$$\frac{dE}{dz} = \alpha' T_2 n(z) E(z) \tag{63}$$

$$0 = [1 - n(z)]/T_1 - T_2 \left(\frac{\wp E}{\hbar}\right)^2 n. \tag{64}$$

These can be combined in a straightforward way using the definition of I and α to give

$$\frac{dI}{dz} = \alpha \frac{I}{1 + I/I_S} \, , \tag{65}$$

where

$$I_S = 1/T_1 T_2 \, . \tag{66}$$

Here, I_S is the traditional saturation power written in atomic units. This is a good starting point for the conversion from atomic to MKS units. Since in practical units, I_S is just $\hbar\nu/\sigma T_1$ where σ is the cross section. Note σ contains T_2 in the form of a bandwidth $\Delta\omega$, where $\Delta\omega = 2/T_2$.

The solution of Eq. (65) is straightforward giving

$$\ell n \frac{I(z)}{I(0)} + \frac{I(z) - I(0)}{I_S} = \alpha z . \tag{67}$$

In the limit of small power, the first term on the left-hand side dominates, giving exponential gain. At high powers, the second term dominates, giving linear growth (i.e., total saturation). Note that if a loss term is included, the field reaches a steady state power at which point the saturated gain (right-hand side of Eq. (3.5) divided by I) equals the loss.

The moment one starts thinking about the solution of CW problems with a degree of profundity greater than that up to now, one runs into enormous conceptual and practical problems. The simplest of these concerns the limits of validity of the monochromatic solution. In Sec. 3 we noted that the atoms can be driven in a periodic fashion at the Rabi flopping frequency. In the present case, this cyclical behavior is damped by the decay processes. However, if the field becomes sufficiently large, the frequency can be much larger than $1/T_2$ or $1/T_1$, and no damping takes place. One can imagine then that the monochromatic solution might become unstable. Although it is relatively straightforward to derive stability equations, their interpretation is ambiguous, unless loss is included. With loss the monochromatic solution does, in fact, become unstable for steady state powers which are 10 times the saturation power. A similar solution of much greater algebraic complexity, exists for the IB medium. In that case, there is little value to pursuing the solution since it is almost always unstable.

The response of a CW amplifier to time varying fields is so involved that general answers seem out of the question. The reason for this is that the fields usually have to be treated statistically. We have, up until now, treated the CW and pulse problems using classical light, which is light with specific amplitudes and phases. The moment statistics are introduced, the classical framework becomes awkward and one's natural inclination is to use quantized fields. Unfortunately, this too has disadvantages since the fields become operators, and the powerful numerical techniques of semi-classical theory can no longer be used.

Thus, for the present, the only approach to this problem with any immediate chance of success is the awkward but numerically calculable classical-statistical description of light. Instead of specifying the exact field input, we specify the moments of the field distribution in the form of correlation functions. The simplest of these is the autocorrelation function of the field $G_1(\tau,z)$ given by

$$G_1(\tau,z) \;=\; \frac{\wp^2}{\hbar^2} \int\limits_{-\infty}^{\infty} d\mu E(\mu,z) E^*(\mu + \tau,z), \qquad (68)$$

or, in shorthand

$$G_1(\tau,z) \;=\; \frac{\wp^2}{\hbar^2} \langle E(0,z) E^*(\tau,z) \rangle . \qquad (69)$$

Higher moments of the correlation function are defined similarly, with quantities like the intensity, intensity squared, etc., replacing the fields. The numerical solution involves using a random number generator to produce an input field with the desired statistics. This is propagated through the amplifier and the evolution of the moments is determined by the suitable integration of the output field.   This process should be repeated until a statistically significant ensemble of inputs is reached.   In practice, the numerical integration is so expensive that one can only hope to guess from one or two examples what the nature of the output will be.

The easiest of all statistical fields to describe is that of noise.   The amplification of noise is, of course, a problem of considerable practical interest, since it leads to parasitic modes, straight amplified spontaneous emission (ASE), and stellar masers.   In addition, in many laser amplifiers, the input light is actually ASE from a nonmode-locked, multimode oscillator.   Noise, which obeys Gaussian statistics, has the property that all of the higher moments of the field can be expressed in terms of $G^{(1)}(\tau, z)$.   For example, the intensity-intensity autocorrelation function obeys the relationship

$$G^{(2)}(\tau, z) = \langle I(\mu, z) I(\mu + \tau, z) \rangle$$

$$= \langle I \rangle^2 + \left\{ G^{(1)}(\tau, z) \right\}^2, \tag{70}$$

where $\langle I \rangle$ is the average power.

The small signal behavior of a random field is not very different from the monochromatic case.   This time, however, we do not assume that the field varies slowly compared to T_2^* (or T_2 in the HB medium).   We allow this since the spontaneous emission has a spectral width of the order of the bandwidth.   In the small signal limit, it is straightforward to reverse the steps given in Sec. 1 to show that

$$\frac{d\tilde{I}(\omega,z)}{dz} \;=\; \tilde{\alpha}(\omega)\tilde{I}(\omega,z). \tag{71}$$

This can be solved in the usual manner to give

$$\tilde{I}(\omega,z) \;=\; \tilde{I}(\omega,0)e^{\tilde{\alpha}(\omega)z}. \tag{72}$$

The gain line $\alpha(\omega)$ is largest at the center, and since it appears in the exponential, it causes the center of the spectrum to grow much more rapidly than the wings. The resulting narrowing of the spectrum is frequently called *Gain Narrowing*. It is straightforward but fairly lengthy to show that, in linear theory, the relationship between $G^{(1)}(\tau,z)$ [which is the Fourier transform of $I(\omega,z)$] and the higher moments is not changed. Thus, the small signal behavior alters the spectrum of the light without changing its Gaussian statistics (i.e., it is still noise). When the amplifying process causes the field to grow large enough to begin to induce nonlinear behavior, two questions arise: first, does the spectrum continue to narrow, and second, does the light remain noise (i.e., does the light statistics change).

The question of the stability of the monochromatic solution plays a key role in the question of narrowing. Monochromatic light has an infinitely narrow spectrum. If it represents an unstable solution, the stable solution, if it exists, must have finite spectral width. Therefore the spectrum cannot narrow indefinitely. The most striking example of finite bandwidth is that for the IB medium in which a large monochromatic (or quasi-monochromatic) wave burns a narrow hole in the region of the center of the

line. This greatly reduces the gain near the center so
that the wings of the spectrum have more gain than the
center. This causes *Saturation Broadening* of the spectrum.
Note that in the HB medium and also in MB cases, the Rabi
flopping effect can cause broadening.

It is not a simple matter to determine what happens to
the photon statistics when rebroadening occurs. Investiga-
tions to date have strongly suggested that they become dis-
tinctly non-Gaussian, but there is little one can say of a
precise nature. Figure 8 gives an example of the evolution
of the intensity and field from noise to gain narrowed
noise and finally to the saturation rebroadened field.
Note the smoothing out of the field in the time domain
which is the equivalent of narrowing in frequency. Thus
the autocorrelation function in the second case is wider
than the first, corresponding to a narrower spectrum. The
evolution from the second to third picture involves primarily the amplitude. There is little change in the phase.
This evolution in amplitude alone is in itself a demonstration of a change in the statistics which is basically a
measure of the relative amounts of amplitude and frequency
fluctuations in the light. It is beyond the scope of these
lectures to investigate the IB noise amplifier in greater
detail. It is unfortunate that the topic is so very difficult since the stellar maser is almost certainly IB, and is
a subject of considerable current interest. We note only a
few salient features. The output from such an amplifier is
a train of pulses that is irregular in two ways. First,
the pulses are nonperiodic, differing in amplitude, width,
and spacing. The pulse train continues to evolve as more
amplifying medium is encountered so there is no asymptotic

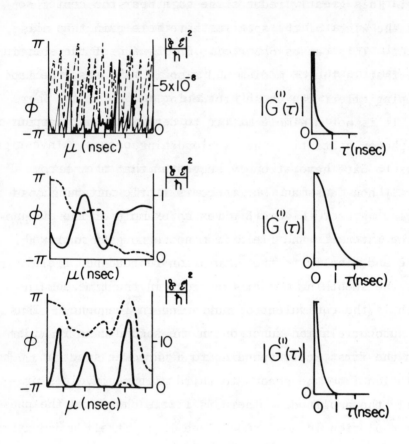

Fig. 8. *Evolution of noise in an amplifier. Last case is*
saturation rebroadened light and has lost its
noise-like character.

configuration. Unlike noise, however, there is an underlying cause-and-effect relationship in the location and
size of the pulses due to the saturation and repopulation
effects that determine whether the individual pulses have
gain. It is in the consequences of this physics that the
most sensitivie test of non-Gaussian statistics can be made.
For example, it is very improbable in the IB amplifier that

two large pulses would be close together since the first
uses up the gain needed to sustain the second. In noise,
the relative size and location of pulses is uncorrelated.
This "anticoincidence" effect is relatively easy to check
and shows up systematically in the computer runs. There
has not yet, however, been any experimental verification of
this effect.

The HB noise amplifier is much easier to treat,
especially if there is a small amount of scattering loss
(e.g., dust). This loss need only be large enough to prevent the Rabi flopping effect from causing rebroadening.
Merely because there is a stable zero-bandwidth asymptotic
solution in this limit does not guarantee continual narrowing. We have, however, made exhaustive computer solutions in this case, and have yet to find a solution which
does not narrow. Therefore, we tentatively conclude that
the monochromatic, asymptotic solution is unique. This is
important because it allows for a simple analytic discussion of the photon statistics in this case, a discussion we
turn to now.

In the time domain, a narrow spectrum has the interpretation that both the amplitude and the phase cannot vary
more rapidly than the coherence time T_C which is defined as
the width in time of $G^{(1)}(\tau,z)$. $(1/T_C$ is, in effect, the
spectral width of the line.) As the line narrows, T_C
invariably increases until the condition $T_C \gg T_1, T_2$ is met.
In this case, the fields vary sufficiently slowly that the
rate equation approximation of Sec. 3.2 is valid. Thus,
Eqs. (63) and (64) hold except that E and n are once again
functions of time. Similarly, the solution for $N(\mu,z)$ is
valid as is the resulting equation of motion for the field.

With loss, we have

$$\frac{dI}{dz} = \alpha \frac{I}{1 + I/I_S} - 2\kappa I, \tag{73}$$

which is the exact analogue of the running wave laser equations. The asymptotic solution of this equation is just the constant intensity I_O where

$$I_O = \frac{\alpha - 2\kappa}{2\kappa} I_S. \tag{74}$$

Thus, any initial statistical distribution evolves into one describing a constant amplitude. This is not the same thing, however, as saying that the field becomes monochromatic. Although the amplitude is constant, the phase is not, and thus the light is frequency modulated. In a fully quantized treatment, there is always some amplitude modulation due to spontaneous events. In that case, this largely FM light is described by Poisson-like statistics. The outputs from two typical numerical calculations (i.e., both nonanalytic and nonapproximate) are shown in Fig. 9. The initial amplitude fluctuation is due to the "turning on" of the amplifier. The constant amplitude part later on is the pertinent part with respect to the present discussion. The frequency modulation is apparent in the figure. A straightforward numerical analysis of the fields in this figure reveals that the output cannot possibly be Gaussian noise.

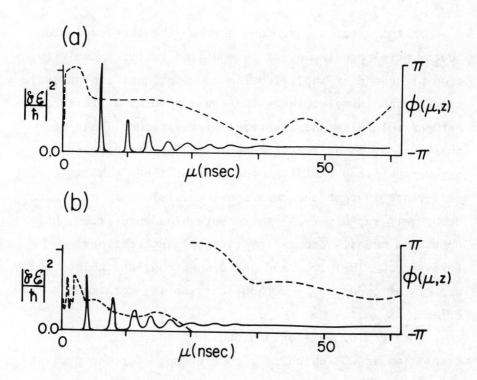

Fig. 9.   Output from a CW homogeneously broadened
          amplifier with random noise input.

3.5.   AMPLIFICATION ON VIBRATIONAL-ROTATIONAL TRANSITIONS

In this section, we consider how the two-level atom theory developed in Sec. 2 is modified to treat the situation presented by amplification on rotational-vibrational transitions in molecules. There are several differences between molecular and electronic transitions. Many of these are of minor consequence in the amplifier, and are not worthwhile pursuing at the present time. The important difference is that the rotational collisions in molecules occur very rapidly $(\sim T_2)$. Pressure broadened (i.e., HB) operation usually occurs in practical applications (pressures ≥ 10 Torr), and one cannot consider pulses which are of the order of T_2 without considering rotational effects as well.

In Fig. 10, we show a picture of the $00^{\circ}1 \rightarrow 10^{\circ}0$ transition in CO_2 which is a good example for the present discussion. The energy is initially stored in the upper vibrational rotational states. As the energy is extracted from the single lasing level, the rotational levels repopulate the active state via rapid collisions. Thus, these collisions appear in the equations in the form of a pump term similar to the ones in Eqs. (61) and (62). However, in this case since there is only a finite amount of energy in the rotational states, the pump can saturate. The simplest terms that can be introduced to describe saturable pump are of the form

$$\dot{n} = (N-n)/T_1' - \ldots \tag{75}$$

$$\dot{N} = (n-N)/T_1'' - \ldots, \tag{76}$$

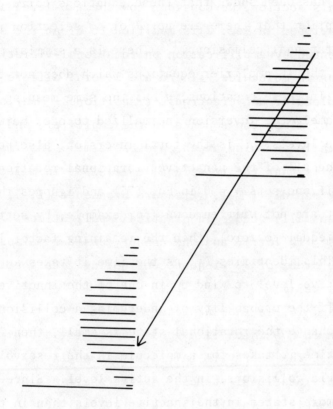

*Fig. 10.   Schematic representation of a vibrational-
            rotational transition.*

where we have not written all of Eq. (75) since the
remaining terms are identical to those in the HB equation
(28). It has been shown that these equations correspond to
the assumption that there are no ΔJ or Δm selection rules
in the rotational collisions.[17] There is a similar modification of the IB amplifier equations which does not concern
us here. In these equations, n has the same meaning as
before, namely the inversion (normalized to one) between
the active levels. N is the total inversion, also normalized, among all of the nonactive vibrational-rotational
states. If one sets $N = 0$ in Eq. (75) and ignores the
terms that are not written down (for example, by setting
the field equal to zero), then the remaining factor is
$-n/T_1'$. This identifies T_1' as the time it takes an atom
in the active level to wind up in one of the inactive
levels. If the probability of undergoing a collision which
does not change the rotational state is small, then T_1'' is
just the time it takes for a molecule in the reservoir to
wind up, via collisions, in the active level. Since there
are many more states in the inactive levels than in the
active level, this second time is considerably slower than
T_1'. In particular

$$\frac{T_1''}{T_1'} = \frac{\text{\# molecules in the reservoir}}{\text{\# molecules in the active levels}} , \qquad (77)$$

where the number of molecules is measured in zero field.
This can be shown directly with a simple calculation of the
stored energy. In the rate equation approximation of Sec.
3, the pulse varies little in a time T_2 and therefore it
varies little in the times T_1' and T_1'' as well. Hence one

gets

$$\frac{\partial I}{\partial z} = \alpha I n \tag{78}$$

$$\dot{n} = (N-n)/T_1' - T_2 I n \tag{79}$$

$$\dot{N} = (n-N)/T_1''. \tag{80}$$

These equations, in spite of their simplicity, are not soluble analytically. To get the conservation of energy here, one substitutes Eq. (80) into Eq. (79) and then substitutes the result into Eq. (78) to get

$$\frac{\partial I}{\partial z} = -\frac{\alpha}{T_2}\left(\dot{n} + \frac{T_1''}{T_1'}\,\dot{N}\right). \tag{81}$$

The time integral of Eq. (81) which gives the energy is now straightforward. As with all rate equations, n and N go to zero (i.e., equal populations) as $t \to \infty$. Then

$$\frac{dT}{dz} = \frac{\alpha}{T_2}\left(1 + \frac{T_1''}{T_1'}\right) = 2\alpha'\left(1 + \frac{T_1''}{T_1'}\right). \tag{82}$$

The stored energy (twice this quantity) is thus augmented over the two-level atom case by the ratio of T_1'' to T_1' which confirms the relationship in Eq. (77).

There is another useful calculation that can be performed using these equations. For I = constant, then Eq. (79) and Eq. (80) are simple differential equations

that can be solved in the usual manner. This allows us to
calculate the energy extracted as a function of time,
namely

$$\frac{d}{dz} \int_0^\mu d\mu' I(\mu',z) = \frac{\alpha}{T_2} \left\{ 1 - n(\mu,z) + \frac{T_1''}{T_1'} \right.$$

$$\left. \times \ [1 - N(\mu,z)] \right\}. \tag{83}$$

From this, we can calculate the amount of energy
remaining in the levels by subtracting Eq. (83) from
Eq. (82). The fraction of energy that is extracted from
the molecules as a function of time is then

$$f(\mu) = \frac{[1-n(\mu)] + \frac{T_1''}{T_1'} [1-N(\mu)]}{1 + T_1''/T_1'}. \tag{84}$$

This quantity is shown in Fig. 11 for several different
powers. Note that as the power increases, the part of the
energy that is in the active levels, $1/(1 + T_1''/T_1')$, is
extracted with an ever increasing rate. The rest of the
energy is limited by the kinetic processes and can be
extracted no more rapidly than T_1'', no matter how large the
field gets.

The numerical calculations of the development of the
pulse show the effects of this dominance of the kinetic
processes. In Fig. 12, we show enhancements for various
different pulse widths (we actually change T_1' and T_1'',
keeping the pulse width constant at $\hat{t}_I = 21.6 \ T_2^*$, but the
effect is the same). Note here that the pulse widths are

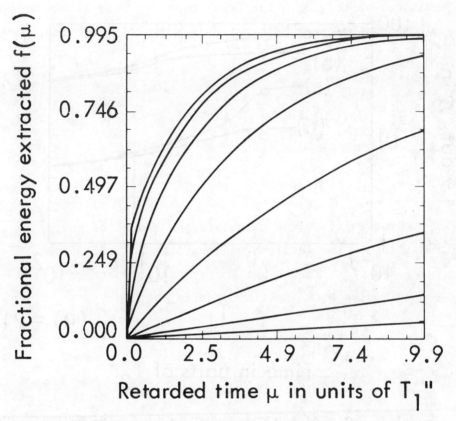

*Fig. 11.   Extracted energy from a molecular system vs
retarded time μ. The higher curves represent
greater optical intensities interacting with the
active levels. The top curve represents limiting
behavior and illustrates the time delay due to
the finite rate of molecular relaxation. The
time scale of the transfer is given essentially
by* T_1''.

measured for the function $I(\mu)$, hence the subscript on $\hat{t}_I$.
One sees large enhancements for widths $\gg T_1'$ and a drop
off as the time T_1' is increased (or equivalently, as the
width is decreased). The reason for this is that the energy
extraction is limited by the rotational kinetics, and if
the pulse is too short, it cannot extract energy from the

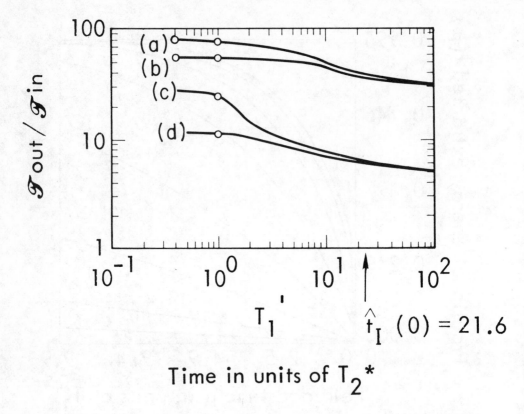

Fig. 12. *Ratio of the pulse energy out to the pulse energy
in, i.e., enhancement, vs T_1' for pulses with an
initial width given by $\hat{t}_I(0) = 21.6$. The parameters are given as follows: (a) $\theta(0) = \pi$, T_1''/T_1'
= 10; (b) $\theta(0) = \pi$, $T_1''/T_1' = 1$; (c) $\theta(0) = 2\pi$,
$T_1''/T_1' = 10$; (d) $\theta(0) = 2\pi$, $T_1''/T_1' = 1$. Complete extraction only occurs for T_1' significantly
less than $\hat{t}_I(0)$. All times are in units of T_2^*.*

rotational states. In Fig. 13, we show the widths of the
output intensity I (input = 10.6) as a function of the time
constants T_1' and T_1''. When these are long, the pulse
behaves as in a two-level system, with considerable narrowing. With shorter times, the reservoir becomes important and typically gives a broadening effect as in A and C.

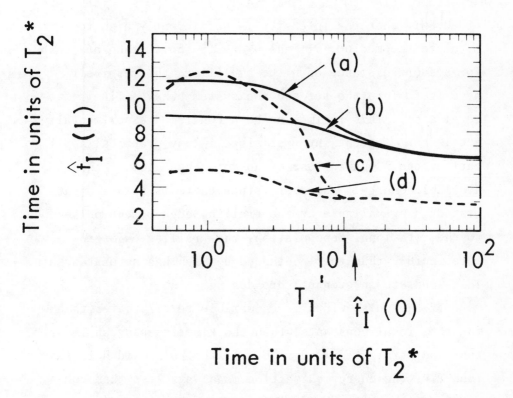

Fig. 13.   *Output-pulse width* $\hat{t}_I(L)$ *vs relaxation time* T_1'.
*The fixed parameters for the curves are as fol-
lows: (a)* $\theta(0) = \frac{1}{2}\pi$, $T_1''/T_1' = 1$; *(b)* $\theta(0) = \frac{1}{2}\pi$,
$T_1''/T_1' = 1$; *(c)* $\theta(0) = 2\pi$, $T_1''/T_1' = 10$; *(d)*
$\theta(0) = 2\pi$, $T_1''/T_1' = 1$. *In all cases* $\hat{t}_I(0)$
= 10.8 T_2^*. *Notice that curves (a) and (c)
actually correspond to a pulse broadening as a
result of the influence of the reservoir. All
times are in units of* T_2^*.

In B and D, the population in the reservoir is small
($T_1' = T_1''$), and one sees that there is a narrowing effect
if the width is greater than T_1'' (this is beginning to show
up in curve C as well for very short times).

The transient aspects of the molecular amplifier can
then be summarized in a fairly straightforward way. The

development is dominated basically by the pulse width, provided only that the intensity is sufficiently high to
saturate the medium. If the width is short, then at least
for a short distance down the amplifier, the reservoir
never gets into the act and the system behaves like a two-
level atom. This regime has been confirmed experimentally,
but is not of great interest since in any practical application, one is making use of no more than ~10% of the
available energy. Moreover, since there is always unsaturated gain available at the trailing edge of the pulse due
to the rotational repopulation, the trailing edge grows
more rapidly than the leading edge which has saturated gain.
This leads to an eventual broadening.

     If the pulse width is comparable to or greater than
the rotational constants, then the kinetics play an important and straightforward role. If the pulse width is less
than T_1'', the energy extraction is always less than complete and the pulse tends to broaden. If the width is
greater than T_1'', then, for large powers, one can extract
half of the energy which is the limit imposed by the lack
of atomic coherence. In this regime, the pulses narrow,
but never become any shorter than T_1''.

     Because of the limitations of the rotational kinetics,
the molecular amplifier has a property that is different
from other models, namely the existence in the HB limit of a
stable unique asymptotic pulse shape whose time scales and
features are determined by the medium kinetics. This waveform is shown in Fig. 14, and is the pulse configuration
towards which all input pulses evolve. The waveform has
two features: an initial short pulse with a width slightly
shorter than T_2, and a long pulse with an exponentially

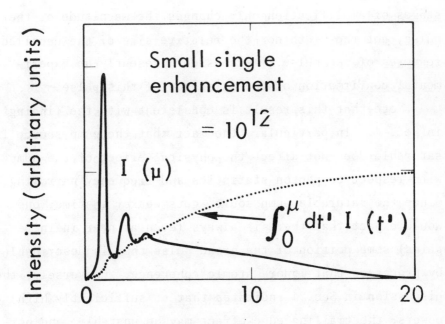

Fig. 14. Intensity I(μ) vs retarded time μ for the charac-
          teristic pulse envelope developed in a high-gain
          amplifier is given by the solid line. The dashed
          contour is the integrated energy of the pulse as
          a function of retarded time μ. The parameters
          corresponding to the calculation are: small
          signal enhancement = 10^{12}, $T_2^* = 1$, $T_2 = 1$,
          $T_1' = 2$, and $T_1'' = 10$.

falling edge whose shape is given by $\exp(-\mu/T_1'')$. The
energy in these two features is partitioned exactly between
the amount in the active level initially (short piece) and
the amount in the other levels (long piece). If the gain
is sufficiently large, then for all but very peculiar input
pulses, this is the waveform at the output. Adding more

stages of amplification only changes the magnitude of the pulse, not the width nor the relative size of the detailed features of the pulse. We consider presently an experimental confirmation of the existence of this pulse.

Note that this result is consistent with the findings in Sec. 4. In particular, the fact that the pump source is saturable does not affect the physical effect of the pump with respect to photon statistics and frequency narrowing. Since the saturable pump source gets weaker in time, one would expect that there is always (even at near infinite gains) some portion of the broad pulse that is describable by processes that ignore atomic coherence. Conversely, the discussion in Sec. 4 indicates that at sufficiently high powers, the trailing edge effect may be unstable, and portions of the broad component might break up into short pulses. We have not been able to continue the numerical calculation into that regime.

As in Sec. 4, one can use rate equation calculations to describe the pulse once the coherent transient has died away. Because of its importance in the molecular amplifier, we give this the name *Maximum Energy Extraction Calculation*. In particular, we consider Eqs. (78) - (80) in the limit that the power becomes very large. In that case, since the left-hand side of Eq. (78) must be finite, it follows that n must be very small, and we take it to be zero. It follows then than $\dot{n}$ must also be zero. We can, accordingly, neglect $\dot{n}$ in Eq. (81) and can directly substitute $\dot{N} = N/T_1''$. To calculate N, one just ignores n in Eq. (80) to get

$$N = \exp[-\mu/T_1'']. \tag{85}$$

Substitution as indicated into Eq. (81) gives

$$\frac{\partial I}{\partial z} = \frac{\alpha}{T_1 T_2} \exp[-\mu/T_1''] . \tag{86}$$

Since the right-hand side of Eq. (86) is independent of both I and z, it is trivial to integrate that equation. One gets

$$I(\mu, z) = I(\mu, 0) + \frac{\alpha z}{T_1 T_2} \exp[-\mu/T_1''] . \tag{87}$$

In the limit of a high gain amplifier, αz is large and the second term in the right-hand side of Eq. (87) dominates. This is precisely what happens in the long pulse part of the asymptotic waveform. Detailed comparison shows that the numerical calculation gives almost precisely an exponential fall-off with a time constant T_1''.

This type of calculation is particularly simple and we continue to exploit it throughout the rest of this section. Note that if one wishes to consider much more complicated models than those here, one could always get the asymptotic waveform in this fashion and avoid the complexities of a complete numerical calculation.

The existence of an asymptotic pulse shape is particularly disturbing from the standpoint of fusion applications (Chaps. 7-9) since it suggests that there is little or no flexibility in the output. In particular, at the pressures that are currently achievable (~3 atm), the output pulses may still be too long to be useful (~1 nsec).

One can shorten the pulses by the simple expedient of operating on more than one rotational line at the same time. Since the probability that a collision excites the molecule to an active level is directly proportional to the number of active levels, the rate of extraction (in turn, directly proportional to this probability) is augmented by an increase in the number of active levels.

We can use the energy extraction calculation to show this in a straightforward way. We assume that the number of molecules in the active states remains small, so that collisions that take the molecule from one active level to another can be neglected. For simplicity, we also take T_1' and T_1'' to be the same for each pair of levels. It is straightforward, but notationally tedious, to consider the more general case. We can then expand the set of Eqs. (78) - (80) to include K pulses operating on levels $k = 1, K$ with inversions n_k and an inversion N between the inactive levels, i.e.,

$$\frac{\partial I_k}{\partial z} = g I_k n_k \tag{88}$$

$$\dot{n}_k = (N - n_k)/T_1' - T_2 I_k n_k \tag{89}$$

$$\dot{N} = \sum_{k=1}^{K} (n_k - N)/T_1''. \tag{90}$$

Again one sets $n_k = 0$, $\dot{n}_k = 0$ and substitutes Eq. (89) into Eq. (88). This gives

$$\frac{\partial I_k}{\partial z} = \frac{g}{T_2 T_1'} \, N(\mu), \tag{91}$$

where

$$N(\mu) = \exp[-\mu K/T_1']. \tag{92}$$

The slow component of the asymptotic pulse is proportional
to $N(\mu)$ and is now shorter by the amount K than it would be
if only one level were used.

This type of a multiple line approach can be used with
simultaneous operation on both the P and R branches of CO_2.
In that case, it turns out that one can increase the
extracted energy from one-half to two-thirds of the stored
energy. For the HF amplifier, we see even more evidence
of the desirability of extraction of energy on more than
one line. This is revealed by experiments we discuss now.

HF Comparison with Experiment

In a recent experiment at Lawrence Livermore Laboratories,[7] a relativistic electron gun was used to initiate
an explosive reaction in an H_2, NF_3 mixture. The excited
HF amplified an input "pulse" which consisted of a low
power single-mode HF oscillator that passed continuously
through the reaction chamber but was amplified only in the
duration of the reaction. The experiment was far from
"clean" in the sense that the amplifier environment was
hard to reproduce and very nonuniform. In addition, there

were shock waves and X-rays that interfered greatly with
diagnostics and performance.

Within the experimental error, one key result emerged,
namely that the output from the amplifier was an asymptotic
waveform of precisely the sort indicated earlier in this
section. Representative samples of the output waveforms
are given in Fig. 15. The differences in the waveforms are
largely instrumental, and are well within the experimental
error. One sees a short, powerful, but low energy initial
spike that is followed by a broad pulse with much greater
energy. The shape is independent of any manipulations that
could be performed on the system. The gain was always
sufficiently large (~300 db of amplification) that the
output pulse was far into the saturation regime. This
result would seem to be an *a priori* confirmation of the
theoretical prediction. There is, however, a significant
difference between the present circumstances and the case
in CO_2 which prevents a straightforward comparison of that
theory with experiment. In the previous calculation, the
pump processes were taken to have preceded the pulse,
whereas in HF the pumping is simultaneous with the pulse.
This turns out to have a significant effect on the theoretical prediction. In particular one does not generally
expect to see as large a coherent transient as is seen
experimentally.

The presence of a time varying pump is introduced in a
straightforward way into the equations. In particular
Eq. (75) must be generalized further so that

$$\dot{n} = [\lambda(\mu) - n]/T_1 + (N-n)/T_1' - \ldots, \qquad (93)$$

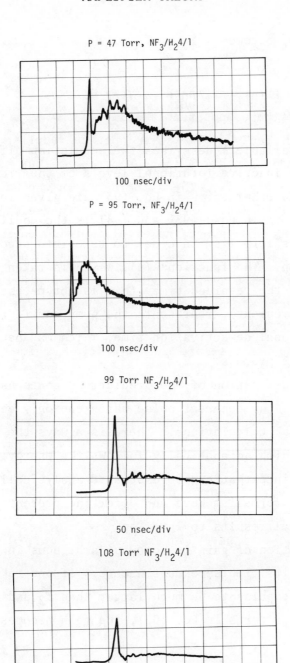

Fig. 15.   *Representative samples of the output waveforms for an HF amplifier.*

and Eq. (76) becomes

$$\frac{dN}{d\mu} = [\lambda(\mu) - N]/T_1 + (n-N)/T_1''. \tag{94}$$

Again the variable N describes the population difference between the inactive rotational levels of the vibrational states. The other terms in Eq. (93) are given in Eq. (28). The first term in Eqs. (93) and (94) is the modification of the previous formalism in order to take into account a time varying pump. The function $\lambda(\mu)$, which is taken to be a function of the retarded time (this is not necessary but it is very convenient), represents the pump and T_1 represents the vibrational de-activation time, which may be either a V-V or a V-T process.

The modification of the predictions concerns the existence of the coherent pulse which can only be obtained via numerical calculations. There is always the broad component which adiabatically follows the energy extraction process. Since that can be discussed analytically, we develop the formalism here and defer the presentation of the numerical results to later on.

The notion of gain is somewhat ambiguous in this case in view of its time dependent nature. If one takes the width of the pulse to be much larger than T_2 and neglects the nonlinear terms in Eq. (93), the gain becomes

$$g(\mu') = \alpha \int_{-\infty}^{\mu'} d\mu'' \exp[-(\mu'-\mu'')/T_1]\lambda(\mu''). \tag{95}$$

This just the instantaneous inversion times some suitably normalized gain coefficient. We use as a convention here that when we refer to a specific value of the gain (g_o), we mean the maximum (in time) of the function $g(\mu)$.

The energy extraction calculation involves taking the time variation of both the field and the inversion to be slow in comparison to T_2. The equations of motion can then be considerably simplified to give

$$\frac{\partial n}{\partial \mu} \;=\; [\lambda(\mu) - n]/T_1 + (N-n)/T_1' - T_2 I n \tag{96}$$

$$\frac{\partial N}{\partial \mu} \;=\; [\lambda(\mu) - N]/T_1 + (n-N)/T_1'', \tag{97}$$

where the field evolution is described by Eq. (78).

In the limit of total saturation, I becomes large and hence n and $\dot{n}$ must go to zero. Taking that limit and substituting Eq. (76) into Eq. (78) one gets

$$\frac{\partial I}{\partial z} \;=\; \frac{2g_o}{T_2}\left(\frac{\lambda(\mu)}{T_1} + \frac{N}{T_1'}\right). \tag{98}$$

Setting $n = 0$ in Eq. (97) allows one to solve for $N(\mu)$ directly giving

$$\frac{\partial I}{\partial z} \;=\; 2g_o I_e(\mu), \tag{99}$$

where

$$I_e(\mu) = \frac{1}{T_1 T_2} \left\{ \lambda(\mu) + \frac{1}{T_1'} \int_0^{\mu} d\mu' \lambda(\mu') \right.$$

$$\left. \times \exp\left[-(\mu-\mu') \left(\frac{1}{T_1} + \frac{1}{T_1''}\right)\right] \right\} . \quad (100)$$

The quantity $I_e(\mu)$ is the energy that is extracted from the amplifier as a function of time under the circumstances in which it is extracted as fast as possible (i.e., in the limit $I \rightarrow \infty$). Note that $I_e(\mu)$ is not dependent on I; hence following the same procedure as that leading to (92), one gets

$$I(\mu,z) = I(\mu,0) + g_o z I_e(\mu). \quad (101)$$

In the limit of large values of $g_o z$, this defines the broad component of the asymptotic pulse. The maximum energy T that can be extracted from the amplifier is given by integrating Eq. (101) to give

$$\frac{dT}{dz} = 2g_o \left[1 + \frac{1}{T_1' \left[\frac{1}{T_1''} + \frac{1}{T_1}\right]}\right] \int_{-\infty}^{\infty} d\mu' \lambda(\mu'). \quad (102)$$

The stored energy is calculated assuming that there are no de-activation processes. This can be easily done by following the same logical sequence leading to Eq. (102) except for setting $T_1 \rightarrow \infty$. The result, expressed as a ratio, is then

$$\frac{\text{Extractable Energy}}{\text{Stored Energy}} = \frac{1 + \dfrac{1}{T_1{}' \left[\dfrac{1}{T_1{}''} + \dfrac{1}{T_1}\right]}}{2\left(1 + \dfrac{T_1{}''}{T_1{}'}\right)}. \qquad (103)$$

The extra factor of two is included since it is conventional to calculate the stored energy as given by the population difference times $\hbar\nu$. Without use of coherent effects, one cannot extract more than half of this energy. The expression in Eq. (103) shows exactly what one expects: $T_1{}''$ is the time it takes to extract the energy from the rotational levels; hence if the de-activation time T_1 is less than $T_1{}''$, one cannot extract all of the available energy. The numerical calculations that are given below suggest that the T_1 process has to be very rapid. Thus, there may be considerable energy lost by operating HF on a single rotational line. This possibility was confirmed in the experiment.

For the numerical calculations presented here, we have chosen the particularly simple case of constant pumping from time 0 to t_p and then zero pumping outside. In Fig. 16, we show a typical output waveform from the numerical calculation along with the function I_e. The output pulse is formed after a distance such that $gL \sim 60$ to 80 and persists without significant change up to the limit at which the numerical calculation becomes unstable ($gL \sim 200$). This range in gains approximately covers those in the experiment. Thus, there is an asymptotic waveform in this case, and except for the coherent response at the

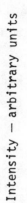
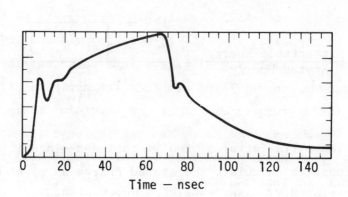

(a)

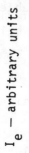
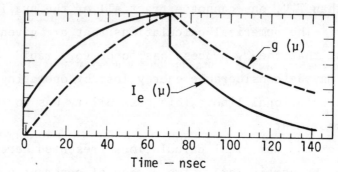

(b)

Fig. 16.   a) Asymptotic pulse waveform: $T_1 = 70$ nsec,
pump pulse duration 70 nsec, $T_2 = 5$ nsec,
$T_2^* = 20$ nsec, $T_1' = 10$ nsec, $T_1'' = 50$ nsec.
(Entire chemical history shown).
b) The function $I_e(\mu)$ shown on the same
scale as the pulse in Fig. 1a.   Also shown
as a broken curve is the function $g(\mu)$.

discontinuity in $\lambda(\mu)$, the broad component does adiabatically follow the energy extraction process given in $I_e(\mu)$. In Fig. 16b the small signal gain of Eq. (95) is shown as well to emphasize that the asymptotic pulse follows $I_e(\mu)$ and not the small signal gain. This point was checked with other forms for $\lambda(\mu)$ and was found to apply in all cases.

The disturbing aspect to the waveform in Fig. 16 is that the coherent pulse on the leading edge is not particularly prominent in contrast to the experimental results. In fact, in general, the coherent pulse does not appear at all. The only case in which one sees a coherent transient is if $\lambda(\mu)$ has a sharply rising (faster than T_2) leading edge as occurs with the present choice of pump. With a fast rise time as a prerequisite, the magnitude of the coherent pulse becomes a function of T_1. This is shown in Fig. 17 where the leading edge of the asymptotic pulse is graphed as a function of T_1. As the de-activation time becomes increasingly small, the coherent pulse gets bigger. This suggests that T_1, although larger than the rotational time T_1', is not very much larger. In particular, it appears that T_1 is less than T_1'', and thus a considerable portion of the available energy is being lost through de-excitation mechanisms before it can be fed into the optical pulse. If one ignores T_1'' compared to T_1 and assumes that $\lambda(\mu)$ varies little in the times T_1' and T_1 (this corresponds to the experimented situation), one finds that

$$I_e(\mu) \cong \frac{1}{T_1 T_2}\left[1 + \frac{T_1}{T_1'}\right]\lambda(\mu). \tag{104}$$

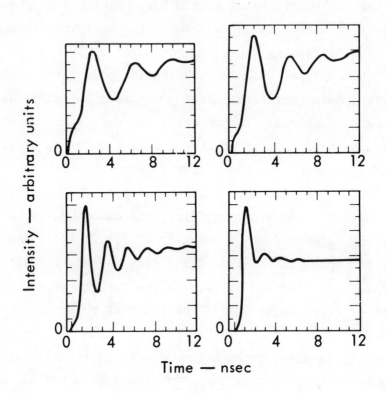

*Fig. 17. Leading edge of the asymptotic pulse waveform
(entire pulse not shown). The times that are
held fixed are: T_2 = 5 nsec, T_2^* = 20 nsec,
T_1' = 10 nsec, T_1'' = 50 nsec. The varied time
constant T_1 is: a) 70 nsec, b) 30 nsec, c) 7
nsec, and d) 1 nsec.*

In other words, the analysis suggests that the experiment depends primarily on chemical pump processes without substantial alteration due to rotational kinetics.

CO -- An Evaluation

Short-pulse amplification in CO can be treated in two parts. First, one can approach it from a purely scientific aspect, and ask whether, for example, the asymptotic pulse could be used to diagnose energy extraction processes. In that context, one would presumably operate on just a single pair of levels in order not to complicate matters, and in that case, the theory outlined earlier is adequate. If one wishes to make a practical short-pulse device, the problems become formidable. In particular, CO is a partially inverted system which virtually rules out appreciable efficiency. Unlike CO_2, however, the energy that is potentially available can actually be retrieved, due to the fact that there are many allowed transitions on only one vibrational mode. In CO_2, there are three vibrational modes and only one transition. Thus, in CO_2 there may be a considerable amount of energy that is hung up in nonusable vibrational modes.

The question of interest here is whether the small part of all of the vibrational energy in CO that can be extracted is greater than that which can be extracted from CO_2. The present efficiency in CO_2 is of the order of 2%. Recent calculations summarized in Ref. 8 suggest that at cryogenic temperatures, one might achieve efficiencies of 10% in CO.

In order to achieve appreciable efficiencies in CO,
one must operate it in a cascade mode with as many R-V
transitions going at the same time as is feasible. This
poses a problem in theoretical development since all of the
conventions in the medium equations used up to now involve
the population differences. When one deals with a cascade,
one must follow the time dependence of each population
separately. The formal development of a theory with all of
the complexities inherent in coherent effects and Doppler
broadening would require still another section. Since we
make no use of this complicated formalism, we develop the
equations in an entirely phenomenological manner.

Using the fact that a light quantum is emitted whenever a transition is made and neglecting atomic coherence
so that the emission and absorption are proportional to the
instantaneous optical power, we can write

$$\frac{1}{\hbar v_v} \frac{dI_v}{dz} = \sigma_v I_v \left(\frac{n_{v+1}}{2J_{v+1} + 1} - \frac{n_v}{2J_{v+1}} \right). \tag{105}$$

Here, n_{v+1} and n_v are the populations of the upper and
lower level rotational-vibrational levels of the transition
$(v+1, J_{v+1}) \rightarrow (v, J)$. The picture of the cascade is shown in
Fig. 18. Note we are specializing the discussion to the
case where the same levels in the rotational set serve as
upper *and* lower states in the cascade. This is not only
simpler theoretically, but also produces short pulses in
the most straightforward manner. In this configuration,
the moleucle can make transitions down many levels in the
cascade at a rate governed by the optical field, which can
be very fast. If different states are used, then there

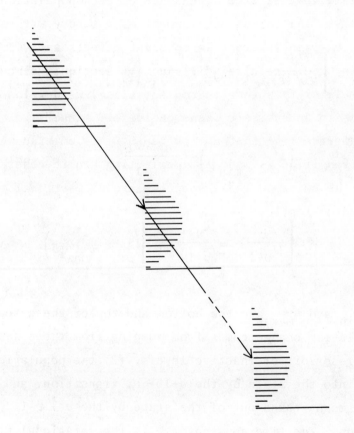

Fig. 18. Schematic representation of a cascade.

must be collision processes that intervene in the cascade
and stretch out the time scale of the maximum-energy-
extraction process determining the asymptotic pulse width.
The factors "$2J+1$" are included since what counts is the
population difference between the magnetic sublevels of the
rotational state.   If we let N_v be the total population of
the inactive levels, then

$$
\dot{n}_v = \left[\frac{N_v}{g(J_v)} - n_v \right] / T_1' + \frac{\sigma_v I_v}{n v_v} \left(\frac{n_{v+1}}{2J_{v+1} + 1} - \frac{n_v}{2J_{v+1}} \right)
$$

$$
\times \left(1 - \delta_{v_{min},v} \right) - \frac{\sigma_{n'} I_{v-1}}{n v_{v-1}}
$$

$$
\times \left[\frac{n_v}{2J_{v+1}} - \frac{n_{v-1}}{2J_{v-1} + 1} \right] \left(1 - \delta_{v_{max},v} \right), \qquad (106)
$$

where v_{min} and v_{max} are the bottom and top of the cascade.
The population change comes from pumping from three sources:
(1) the reservoir of inactive levels, (2) the population
brought into the state by the $v+1 \rightarrow v$, transition, and
(3) the amount taken out of the state by the $v \rightarrow v-1$
transition.   The time constant T_1' is the rotational time
that is taken to be the same for all levels.   The use of
T_1'' here is awkward since there are different ratios of
populations for each level, and since the cumulative change
in J from the top to bottom of the cascade may be very
large.   We use instead the factor $g(J)$ which is the relative population of the inactive and active states.   Since

the rotational states are in equilibrium with the translational motion, one gets directly that

$$g(J) = \frac{\sum_{J=0}^{\infty} \exp[-BJ'(J'+1)/RT](2J'+1)}{\exp[-BJ(J+1)/RT](2J+1)} , \qquad (107)$$

where B is the rotational constant. The equation of motion
of the inactive levels is

$$\dot{N}_v = [g(J_v)n_v - N_v]/g(J_v)T_1'. \qquad (108)$$

We have ignored all V-V and V-T processes since in CO
they are very much slower than the rotational times. In
the duration of a single pulse, the populations are frozen
in, except insofar as they are affected by the optical
fields.

The general solution of these equations of motion,
even with numerical techniques, presents a bewildering
array of possibilities. It is quite common to find, for
example, an absence of gain on certain of the levels unless
other levels are saturated. To discuss a unique situation,
we consider the maximum energy extraction calculation that
defines the asymptotic pulse configuration. First, we
substitute Eqs. (96) and (94) into Eq. (93) to get the
recursive formula

$$\frac{1}{\hbar v_v} \frac{dI_v}{dz} = -(\dot{N}_v + \dot{n}_v) + \frac{1}{\hbar v_{v-1}} \frac{dI_{v-1}}{dz}$$

$$\times (1 - \delta_{v,v\min}). \qquad (109)$$

If one can calculate the population changes, one can in turn get the energy extraction conditions on the various levels by noting that Eq. (109) gives directly

$$\frac{1}{\hbar\nu_\nu} \frac{dI_\nu}{dz} = -\sum_{\nu'=\nu_{min}}^{\nu} (\dot{N}_\nu + \dot{n}_\nu).$$

(110)

As before, the maximum energy extraction calculation is performed in the limit $I_\nu \to \infty$. Since in this case there is no clear *a priori* reason why there should be gain, this means that it is necessary to be careful that the maximum energy extraction is self-consistent. In order that the high powers be available in the first place, it is necessary that the equations represent a growth rather than an attenuation. This is in the nature of a threshold condition, since it is a property of the medium. In order to distinguish it from an ordinary threshold, we call it a *Cascade Extraction Threshold Condition* (CETC). There are several threshold conditions which are discussed shortly. First we must establish the conditions for the calculation of the populations. In the limit of large powers, the populations of the active magnetic sublevels must be the same (i.e., zero inversion). Thus,

$$\frac{n_\nu}{2J_\nu+1} = \frac{n_{\nu'}}{2J_{\nu'}+1}, \quad \nu_{min} \le \nu, \nu' \le \nu_{max}.$$

(111)

Furthermore the total population of all of the active vibrational levels is conserved

$$\sum_{v} (n_v + N_v) \ = \ \sum_{v} N_v \ = \ N. \tag{112}$$

Equations (111) and (112) with (108) are sufficient to
define the time dependence of all of the populations.
There are two necessary and sufficient CETC's for the simultaneous extraction of energy on all of the lines from v_{min}
to v_{max}. The first consists of the condition for extraction of energy in short coherent pulse, and the second is
the condition on the broad pulse that follows.

The short-pulse CETC is somewhat of a guess since we
have eliminated the basic physics that causes it in the
first place. It is reasonable, however, to suppose that if
there is energy available to create the pulse, then it
forms in a manner that is largely similar to the case in
two levels. Since the short pulse response has been
removed from the calculation by making approximations and
by setting $I_v \to \infty$, it is necessary to work some to recover
it. The short pulse is almost entirely a function of the
response of the optical field to the energy that is available in the active levels at retarded time $\mu = 0$. The
first thing to do then is to neglect entirely the role of
the N_v. In that case, the equations represent a generalization of the two-level rate equations whose properties we
already know. In time, they equilibrate the upper and
lower level populations with the value (111). By hypothesis, the inactive levels do not play a role so that the
total number of molecules in the active states is constant,
i.e.,

$$\sum_v n_v(\mu) \;=\; \sum_v n_v(0) \;=\; \sum_v \frac{N_v(0)}{g(J_v)+1}\;. \tag{113}$$

If one sets $T_{CP,v}$ as the energy and integrates Eq. (108) ignoring N_v, one gets

$$\frac{1}{\hbar v_v}\frac{dT_{CP,v}}{dz} \;=\; \sum_{v'=v_{min}}^{v}\,[n_v(0^+) - n_v(0)], \tag{114}$$

where $n_v(0^+)$ is the population after the coherent pulse. This is found by solving Eqs. (113) and (111) together to give

$$\frac{1}{\hbar v_v}\frac{dT_{CP,v}}{dz} \;=\; \sum_{v'=v_{min}}^{v}\left(\left[\frac{(2J_{v'}+1)}{\displaystyle\sum_{v''=v_{min}}^{v_{max}}(2J_{v''}+1)}\right]\right.$$

$$\left.\times\; \sum_{v''=v_{min}}^{v_{max}}\frac{N_{v''}(0)}{g(J_{v''})+1} - \frac{N_{v'}(0)}{g(J_{v'})+1}\right). \tag{115}$$

The first condition, which is called the initiation CETC is that the right-hand side of Eq. (115) be positive for all v. Note that if any term is negative, then the entire scheme is invalid and one must try a different set of J's and v's. The second necessary and sufficient CETC is that the right-hand side of Eq. (108) is positive for all times. There, $\dot{n}_v$ and $\dot{N}_v$ are calculated using

Eqs. (111), (112) and (106). This is a very tedious calculation since the equations are not readily soluble in
closed form. With the nonphysical assumption that the
rotational level populations are equal for all states, the
initiation and time dependent CETC conditions are the same.
Unfortunately CO operation involves a series of P branch
transitions, so that for the case of 10 lines, the
angular momentum difference from top to bottom is 10.
Since the top J's themselves are about 10, the simplifying
assumptions are not at all valid.

   At the present time, work is in progress to evaluate
the CETC's numerically. There is a still simpler CETC
which is a necessary but insufficient condition for the
cascade which is to require only that the total energy
extracted in the transition $v+1 \rightarrow v$ be positive. This was
used in a recent publication[8] in order to evaluate possible
efficiencies. More recent calculations have suggested that
10% is about as good as one can do in CO at cryogenic
temperatures unless one can find a better excitation mechanism. Thus, CO has an ambiguous position in short pulse
studies. It has a better potential efficiency than has
been achieved in practice in other systems. Nonetheless on
paper, other systems (i.e., CO_2) have potentially higher
efficiencies than 10%. It is fitting to end this paper on
this ambiguous point. One can hope that with the tremendous
impetus from the fusion and military programs, questions of
this sort will get straightened out.

3.6.   REFERENCES

The references available to those who work in amplifiers tend to be rather meager. Much of the work remains
unpublished or available only in technical reports. The
following is a partial summary of papers available and per-
sons who have done work in the field from whom material may
be available via private communication.

Section 2

A good source of this material is E. L. Gieszelmann,
Chirped Pulses in Laser Amplifiers thesis, which is pub-
lished as a technical report of the Optical Sciences Center,
University of Arizona.[4] The original work on which this is
based is found in Hopf and Scully.[1] Also useful is
Icsevgi and Lamb.[9] A tutorial overview of amplifier and
attenuator theory is given in in Chapter 13 of the book by
Sargent, Scully, and Lamb.[2]

The work on spatial and etc. transformations is scattered throughout the literature. Reference 10 is of particular interest to the work on reversibility.

Section 3

All of the papers suggested above are pertinent to
this section. In addition, there is the early work on rate
equations by Franz and Nodvik,[11] and Basov et al.[12] Work
was performed by H. Haus (E.E. Dept., MIT) and W. Wagner on
transient pulse development in the HB medium which, to my

knowledge, has never been published . The PB medium has
been discussed extensively by G. Lamb; see his review
article.[13] Work on chirped pulses has been performed by
Carmen and Fleck at LLL that has been reported in The
Fusion Reports. Work on the same subject has been done by
Hahn and Diels[14] and by Treacy.[6] An experimental confirmation of some of the coherent responses was done by P. Hoff
currently at LLL (see Chap. 8) .

Section 4

The simple rate equation calculations are found in
many places, e.g., Ref. 2 and Yariv's text.[15] The noise
amplifier work has been reported in technical meetings and
is currently being prepared for publication by Hopf.[16]

Section 5

The work on molecular amplifiers has been published by
Rhodes and Hopf.[17] The work on CO is published in Ref. 8.
The HF work is currently in preparation (Hopf, Rhodes, and
Krawitz[18]). The notion of using multiple-line extraction
in CO_2 was first brought to the author's attention in a
talk by B. Feldman at the 4th Winter Meeting of the Physics
of Quantum Electronics (1973).

There are several references (19-21) on the subject
of steady state pulses, which are not a subject of these
papers.

APPENDIX A

This appendix contains some of the intermediate steps
in the derivations that are not included in the text.

1. Derivation of the Reduced Wave Equation.

The reduced wave equation (6) follows from Eq. (5)
through an algebraically messy but straightforward series
of steps. One uses the waveform in Eq. (1) and is interested in calculating second derivatives with respect to
time and space. Taking the second time derivative, we see

$$\frac{1}{2} \frac{\partial^2}{\partial t^2} \left\{ E \exp[i(kz-\nu t)] + \text{c.c.} \right\}$$

$$= \frac{1}{2} \left(\frac{\partial^2 E}{\partial t^2} - 2i\nu \frac{\partial E}{\partial t} - \nu^2 E \right) \exp[i(kz-\nu t)] + \text{c.c.} \quad .\text{(A1)}$$

Similarly in the plane wave situation, $\Delta^2 \rightarrow \partial^2/\partial z^2$ and

$$- \frac{1}{2} \frac{\partial^2}{\partial z^2} \left\{ E \exp[i(kz-\nu t)] + \text{c.c.} \right\}$$

$$= - \frac{\partial^2 E}{\partial z^2} + 2ik \frac{\partial E}{\partial z} + k^2 E + \text{c.c.} \quad . \quad\quad\quad \text{(A2)}$$

The left-hand side of Maxwell's equations is found by multiplying Eq. (A1) by $1/c^2$ and adding it to Eq. (A2). There

are three natural groupings of terms; the second derivatives which, by hypothesis, are taken to be small, the
first derivatives which lead to the convective derivative
(see later when the substitution is made), and finally, the
constant term which vanishes because

$$k^2 = v^2/c^2. \tag{A3}$$

The reduction on the right-hand side of Maxwell's
equations is straightforward from an algebraic standpoint,
but involves many logical subtleties. The second derivative of the polarization is

$$\frac{\mu_o}{2} \frac{\partial^2}{\partial t^2} \left\{ P \, \exp[i(kz - vt)] + \text{c.c.} \right\}$$

$$= \frac{\mu_o}{2} \times \left(\frac{\partial^2 P}{\partial t^2} - 2iv \frac{\partial P}{\partial t} - v^2 P \right) \exp[i(kz - vt)] + \text{c.c.} \ . \tag{A4}$$

We are going to neglect all terms on the right-hand
side of Eq. (A4) that involve derivatives of the polarization amplitude. We do this because the polarization is
taken to be "small." This is the tricky aspect to this
calculation. In order to see what this means, it is useful
to digress and treat this point in some detail. Neglecting
the first derivative of P means that

$$\left| \frac{1}{c^2} (2iv) \frac{\partial E}{\partial t} \right| \ \gg \ \left| \mu_o(-2iv) \frac{\partial P}{\partial t} \right| \ , \tag{A5}$$

since we intend to keep the term in the first derivative of
E. If we write (using $\varepsilon_o = 1$) that

$$P = \chi E \tag{A6}$$

then the inequality is the same as demanding that

$$1 \gg \chi. \tag{A7}$$

Since $n^2 = 1+x$, the approximation of small P is the
same as saying that the contributions from the atoms must
involve only a minor perturbation on the index of refraction. At solid state densities (10^{22} atoms/cc), indices
are significantly different from one (i.e., 1.5 or so) and
the approximation breaks down badly. If one wishes to
include the background dispersion into the theory, it must
be done directly in the wave equation (A5). As usual, this
involves replacing $1/c^2$ by n^2/c^2. In the case that one
lets n be a function of frequency, still more care is
called for which is beyond the scope of the present discussion. For atomic densities that are typical for lasing
species (i.e., $\sim 10^{19}$ or smaller), then χ is small and one
can usually ignore the terms involving the derivatives.

If one then substitutes these derivatives back into
Eq. (A5) and neglects the second derivatives in E and all
derivatives in P, then one gets

$$-2ik \frac{\partial E}{\partial z} - \frac{2i\nu}{c^2} \frac{\partial E}{\partial t} = -\mu_o \nu^2 P, \tag{A8}$$

where we have cancelled the rapidly varying exponential terms.

2. Rate Equations.

It is frequently the case that the use of energy conservation forms the basis of rather than, as in the case here, follows as a consequence of the equations for amplification. For completeness, the conventional derivation is shown here. The relationship with the conventions in the text is also given.

Let us take the field to be monochromatic (time independent) with a flux S. The Einstein relations then say that

$$\frac{\partial S}{\partial z} = \sigma(n_a - n_b)S, \tag{A9}$$

where σ is the cross section and n_a and n_b are the populations in the upper and lower levels. The "number of photons" is $S/\hbar\nu$. Thus, the probability of a photon being added to the field is given by $\sigma n_a S/\hbar\nu$ (removed $\equiv n_b$). Since the number of atoms in the upper level is decreased (increased) by this, one has

$$\frac{\partial n_a}{\partial t} = \frac{\sigma n_a S}{\hbar\nu} - \frac{\sigma n_b S}{\hbar\nu} + \lambda_a - n_a/T_1. \tag{A10}$$

Here λ_a is the pump rate to the upper state and $-n_a/T_1$ is the decay rate. We presume there is no pumping to the lower state (this merely simplifies the algebra) and that

the characteristic decay time is the same for both upper
and lower states. Then, since the total population is conserved by the "photon" terms, we have

$$\frac{\partial n_b}{\partial t} = -\frac{\sigma n_a S}{\hbar \nu} + \frac{\sigma n_b S}{\hbar \nu} - n_b/T_1 . \qquad (A11)$$

The equations as they appear in the text are defined
as near as possible depending upon the circumstances, as
the inversion per excited atom (the problems come when the
number of excited atoms are time dependent). To get this
convention, one subtracts Eq. (A11) from Eq. (A10) and
divides by $\lambda_a T_1$. One defines

$$n = \frac{n_a - n_b}{\lambda_a T_1} . \qquad (A12)$$

Then one gets

$$\dot{n} = (1-n)/T_1 - \frac{2\sigma S}{\hbar \nu} n . \qquad (A13)$$

In the atomic units of the text, we have $T_2 I \equiv (2\sigma/\hbar\nu)S$
which casts Eq. (A13) in the form given in the text. Note
that in time, the populations achieve a steady state, so
that $\dot{n}_a = \dot{n}_b = 0$. The algebraic solution of Eq. (A10) and
Eq. (A11) is then straightforward to give

$$\frac{\partial S}{\partial z} = \frac{\alpha S}{1 + S/S_{sat}} , \qquad (A14)$$

where

$$S_{sat} = \frac{\hbar\nu}{2\sigma T_1} .$$

(A15)

The gain, in this case, is given by

$$\alpha = \sigma\lambda_\alpha T_1.$$

(A16)

3.   Derivations of the Energy Formula in the HB Medium.

There are many places in these notes in which certain
properties of the pulse [i.e., $\theta(z)$ in the IB case; $T(z)$
in the HB] obey closed form equations of motion. All of
these involve a certain trick in order to derive them. In
this appendix, we derive the energy law as an example of
how to obtain these results. The derivation of Eq. (40) is
given by substituting Eq. (38) into Eq. (39), namely,

$$\frac{\partial I}{\partial z} = \alpha I \exp\left[-T_2 \int_{-\infty}^{\mu} d\mu' I(\mu',z) \right] ,$$

(A17)

and then integrating in time to get

$$\frac{dT}{dz} = \alpha \int_{-\infty}^{\infty} d\mu I(\mu,z) \exp\left[- \int_{-\infty}^{\mu} d\mu' I(\mu',z) \right] .$$

(A18)

The trick is to note that

$$d\mu I(\mu,z) \;\; = \;\; d\left\{\int_{-\infty}^{\mu} d\mu' I(\mu',z)\right\}.$$

(A19)

So, with the substitution

$$x \;\; = \;\; \int_{-\infty}^{\mu} d\mu' I(\mu',z), \quad x\Big|_{\mu=-\infty} \;\; = \;\; 0, x\Big|_{\mu=+\infty} \;\; = \;\; T,$$

(A20)

Eq. (A18) reduces to

$$\frac{dT}{dz} \;\; = \;\; \alpha \int_{0}^{T} dx e^{-x},$$

(A21)

from which Eq. (40) follows directly.

4. Partial List of Symbols.

The following is a list of symbols used in the notes. Only those symbols used in more than one of the discussions are presented. Standard symbols (e.g., c = speed of light, h = Planck's constant) are taken to be known.

Constant	Meaning and Comments	First Usage (Eq.)
α	Gain constant.	17
α'	Stored energy (two-level atom), closely related to α.	27
$D(T)$	Fourier transform of the unsaturated inhomogeneously broadened line.	14
$E(t,z)$	Total electric field.	1
$E(t,z)$	Complex electric field amplitude.	1
$g(J)$	Fraction of molecules in active rotational state.	88
$g(\mu)$, g_o	Special notation for gain used in context of HF amplifier.	95,99
I	Optical power in "atomic" units; if subscripted by v or k, it means optical power resonant with particular transition.	21
I_S or I_{sat}	Saturation power.	66
$\tilde{I}(\omega,z)$	Power spectrum.	56
k	Wave vector of light.	1
κ	Scattering loss.	6
μ	Retarded time.	32
n	Inversion per atom between upper and lower lasing levels (HB only); if subscripted, it usually means the individual populations. The exception to this latter rule is on p. 136.	26

Constant	Meaning and Comments	First Usage (Eq.)
N	Population difference per molecules in inactive rotational states; if subscripted, the usage parallels that of "n."	76
N	Total number of atoms; if subscripted, it is the total number of atoms in subscripted state. It is never used as an inversion.	88
ν	Light frequency.	1
ω	Atomic frequency.	11
ω_O	Center frequency of inhomogeneous line.	12
$\wp$	Dipole matrix element.	10
ϕ	Phase of the EM field.	3
$P(t,z)$	Complex polarization amplitude.	2
$P(t,z)$	Polarization.	2
$\sigma(\omega)$	Inhomogeneous distribution of atomic frequencies.	15
t	Time.	1
$\hat{t}$	Pulse width [FWHM of field $E(t,z)$].	36
$\hat{t}_I$	Pulse width [FWHM of $I(t,z)$].	
T_2	Phase memory time.	11
T_2^*	Coherent dephasing time.	15
T_1	Atomic lifetime (meaning is used somewhat flexibly in Sec. 3.5).	61

Constant	Meaning and Comments	First Usage (Eq.)
T_1'	Rotational collision time.	75
T_1''	Rotational equilibration time.	76
T	Pulse energy in atomic units.	22
T	Time component in inhomogeneous susceptibility $\chi(T,t,z)$.	18
$W(\omega,t,z)$	Inversion per atom at frequency ω in an inhomogeneous line.	10
$\chi(T,t,z)$	Susceptibility per atom of inhomogeneously broadened line.	18

APPENDIX B

In this appendix, we derive the equation (25) which describes conservation of energy in the two-level atom medium. Evaluating the equation of motion (24) for the nonlinear susceptibility at $T = 0$, we find

$$\frac{\partial \chi(0,t,z)}{\partial t} = -\frac{\wp^2}{2\hbar^2} \int_{-\infty}^{t} dt' \exp[-(t-t')/T_2]$$

$$\times \{E(t,z)E^*(t',z)\chi(-t+t',t',z)$$

$$+ E^*(t,z)E(t',z)\chi(t-t',t',z)\}, \tag{B1}$$

which can be rewritten using the symmetry relationship of the susceptibility

$$\chi(T,t,z) = \chi^*(-T,t,z), \tag{B2}$$

to give

$$\frac{\partial \chi(0,t,z)}{\partial t} = -\frac{\wp^2}{2\hbar^2} \Bigg\{ \Bigg[E^*(t,z) \int_{-\infty}^{t} dt' \; (t',z)$$

$$\exp[-(t-t')/T_2]\chi(t-t',t',z) \Bigg]^*$$

$$+ E^*(t,z) \int_{-\infty}^{t} dt' E(t',z)\exp[-(t-t')/T_2]$$

$$\times \chi(t-t',t',z) \Bigg\} . \tag{B3}$$

The right-hand side of Eq. (B3) is just the integral that
appears in the equation of motion of the electromagnetic
pulse, Eq. (7).   By direct substitution then,

$$\frac{\partial \chi(0,t,z)}{\partial t} = -\frac{1}{\alpha}\frac{\wp^2}{2\hbar^2}\left[E(t,z)\left(\frac{\partial E^*}{\partial z} + \frac{1}{c}\frac{\partial E^*}{\partial t}\right)\right.$$

$$\left. + E^*(t,z)\left(\frac{\partial E}{\partial z} + \frac{1}{c}\frac{\partial E}{\partial t}\right)\right].\qquad (B4)$$

The right-hand side can be rewritten directly using
the definition of I.   This gives

$$\frac{\partial I}{\partial z} + \frac{1}{c}\frac{\partial I}{\partial t} = -2\alpha\,\frac{\partial \chi(0,t,z)}{\partial t}\ .\qquad (B5)$$

This is the relationship, Eq. (25), expressing conservation
of energy.   Using the definitions of α, Eq. (23), and of χ,
Eq. (18), one gets

$$\frac{1}{\hbar\nu}\left[\left(\frac{c\varepsilon_o}{2}\right)\frac{\hbar^2}{\wp^2}\right]\left\{\frac{\partial I}{\partial z} + \frac{1}{c}\frac{\partial I}{\partial t}\right\} = -\frac{N}{2}\frac{\partial}{\partial t}\int$$

$$d\omega\sigma(\omega)W(\omega,t,z).\qquad (B6)$$

The term in the square brackets is the conversion from I to
ordinary units, so that the left-hand side of Eq. (B6) has
the interpretation of the change in the number of photons.
The right-hand side is just the change in number of atoms.
The factor of two comes from the fact that when an atom
goes from the upper to the lower state, the inversion

(single atom) goes from +1 to -1, i.e., changes by a factor
of two.

APPENDIX C

The techniques for programming the amplifier equations
of motion are now fairly well known. For the beginner,
however, there is one pitfall that must be avoided, namely
that the differential equation (31) must not be taken
literally. Rather it must be considered in the time-
retarded frame as in Eq. (33). Specifically, noticing that
in going from z to $z + G$, that one also goes from
t to $t+G/c$, one might choose a time scale grid of G/c.
Such a scale causes considerable difficulty and leads to
potential sources of programming inefficiency.

As was shown in Sec. 2, the convective derivative
merely redefines the zero in time from one step to the
next. Thus, the proper time gridding is G/c, $G/c+H$,
$G/c+2H$, ... etc. In practice, it is never necessary to
keep track of the G/c term. If one uses an array $E(I)$,
then the $I = 1$ term just represents the point $\mu = 0$
(i.e., $t = G/c$) at all spatial steps. The grid in the spatial domain is shown pictorially in Fig. 19.

The results presented in this chapter have been
obtained by a second-order predictor-corrector method, with
trapezoidal rule methods for the integrals. This generally
results in an accuracy of 5% which is sufficient for most
cases. The greatest source of inaccuracy (other than
instabilities in the program which we discuss shortly) is
in the normalization of $D(T)$ and the specification of the

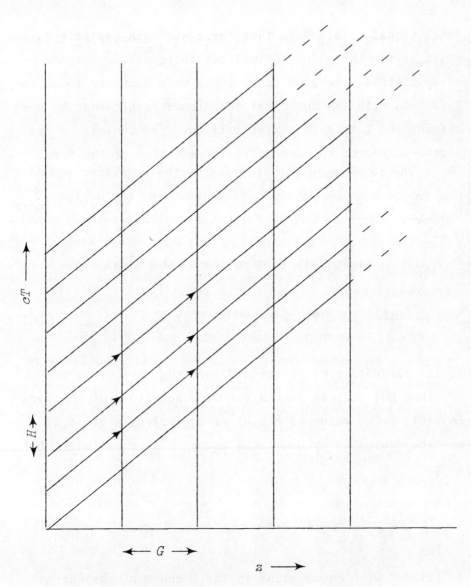

*Fig. 19. This figure represents the direction in the
space-time coordinate system used in the
predictor-corrector routine in finding the
electric field.*

small signal gain. Note that there are both explicit integrals as for the gain and implicit integrals as in the
normalization. In each case, it is more accurate to do the
integrals with the numerical techniques rather than by specifying the integrals analytically or from tables. A predictor-corrector routine solves an equation of the form

$$\frac{dy}{dz} = F(z,y).\tag{C1}$$

The equations solved here are of the form

$$\frac{\partial E(\mu,z)}{\partial z} = \alpha'P(\mu,z).\tag{C2}$$

If the retarded time is gridded such that μ = 0, H, $2H$, ...
NH, then Eq. (C2) is just a set of N equations of the form
Eq. (C1). The value of $P(\mu,z)$ or equivalently $\chi(T,t,z)$
must be evaluated by numerical means. The equation of the
form

$$\frac{\partial \chi(P,\mu,z)}{\partial \mu} = F(T,t,z),\tag{C3}$$

is gridded with equal steps in the T and t dimensions as
shown in Fig. 20. With this gridding, Eq. (C3) consists of
N (not $2N$ because of symmetry relations in the T dimension)
simultaneous equations of the form of Eq. (C1) and is
solved by the same methods. The gridding allows for a
great economy in specifying the right-hand side of Eq. (C3)
since the integrals can be written in recursive form. Note
also that the right-hand side of Eq. (C2) and Eq. (C3) are

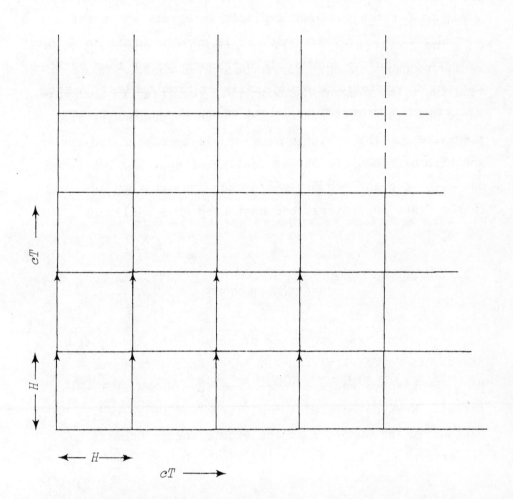

Fig. 20. This figure represents the direction in a space-time system used by the predictor-corrector routine in finding the susceptibility. The spatial coordinate is constant (i.e., this is all taking place at a fixed position z).

related (see Appendix B) and do not need to be separately calculated.

The greatest difficulty in running the numerical code is the tendency of Eq. (C3) to become unstable. This results in the program "blowing up," resulting in absurdly large numbers. This can only be cured by decreasing the step size H. The criterion for stability depends on the specific problem. If one is dealing with atomic coherence, one must keep the product $\wp H E/\hbar$ much smaller than one, and in the "rate" equations, one must keep $H T_2 I$ small.

ACKNOWLEDGMENTS

This work was supported principally by the United States Air Force, Kirtland Air Force Base (Air Force Weapons Laboratory) and Air Force Cambridge Research Laboratories. Work on molecular amplifiers was performed in part under the auspices of the Atomic Energy Commission (Livermore).

REFERENCES

1. F. A. Hopf and M. O. Scully, Phys. Rev. 179 399 (1969).

2. M. Sargent III, M. O. Scully, and W. E. Lamb, Jr., *Laser Physics*, Addison-Wesley Publishing Co., Reading, Mass. (1974). Chap. 13.

3. R. H. Dicke, Phys. Rev. 93, 99 (1954).

4. E. L. Gieszelmann, Ph.D. dissertation, University Microfilms, Ann Arbor, Michigan (1973). (Also, an Optical Sciences Technical Report 80, University of Arizona.)

5. S. L. McCall and E. L. Hahn, Phys. Rev. 183, 457 (1969).

6. E. B. Treacy, Physics Letters 28A, 34 (1968). See also Annals of N. Y. Academy of Sciences 168, 400 (1970).

7. B. Krawitz, Ph.D. dissertation, University Microfilms, Ann Arbor, Michigan (1973).

8. F. A. Hopf, Optics Comm. 9, 38 (1973).

9. A. Icsevgi and W. E. Lamb, Jr., Phys. Rev. 185, 517 (1969).

10. F. A. Hopf and J. Goldstein, Optics Comm., to be published. The discussion in the text is somewhat over-simplified. A proper discussion is given in this reference.

11. L. M. Franz and J. Nodvik, J. Appl. Phys. 34, 2346 (1963).

12. N. G. Basov, R. V. Ambartsumyan, V. S. Zuev, P. G. Kryukov, and V. S. Letokhov, Zh. Eksp. i Teor. Fiz 50, 23 [Eng. transl: Soviet Phys. JETP 23, 16 (1966)].

13. G. L. Lamb, Jr., Rev. Mod. Phys. 43, 99 (1971).

14. E. L. Hahn and J. P. Diels, Phys. Rev. A8, 1084 (1973).

15. A. Yariv, *Introduction to Optical Electronics*, Holt, Rinehart and Winston (1971).

16. F. A. Hopf, to be published.

17. C. K. Rhodes and F. A. Hopf, Phys. Rev. $\underline{A8}$, 912 (1973).

18. F. A. Hopf, C. K. Rhodes and B. Krawitz, to be
     published.

19. J. P. Wittke and P. J. Warter, J. Appl. Phys. $\underline{35}$, 1668
     (1964).

20. F. T. Arecchi and R. Bonifaccio, IEEE J. Quantum
     Electron., $\underline{QE-1}$, 169 (1965).

21. J. A. Armstrong and E. Courtens, IEEE J. Quantum
     Electron., $\underline{QE-4}$, 411 (1968).

PROPAGATION OF HIGH ENERGY LASER
BEAMS IN THE ATMOSPHERE
Charles B. Hogge

4.1. INTRODUCTION

When laser radiation is transmitted through the
atmosphere, numerous physical processes can occur that,
generally speaking, alter the nature of the beam. When
the power in the beam is low, the processes tend to be
linear in nature. At high powers, new processes are found
to occur. Depending on the specific application, these
processes may limit the usefulness of the laser system.

In this chapter I discuss these general topics con-
cerning propagation of high energy laser beams in the
atmosphere. The first subject is atmospheric turbulence
(Sec. 4.2). This phenomenon affects both high and low
power beams. A brief introduction to the atmospheric
effects that are the source of optical degradations is
given. I then describe briefly the theoretical implications of the propagation of focused beams, and describe
the experimental observations which have been made

specifically on this aspect of propagation in a turbulent atmosphere.

The second subject is the thermal blooming of high energy laser beams (Sec. 4.3). Particular emphasis is placed in 10.6 μm systems and the kinetic processes associated with the absorption of this wavelength in the atmosphere. A discussion of the current status of theoretical calculations is given and examples of the parameter dependencies of the phenomena is shown. The propagation of pulsed laser systems is discussed and results of some recent work presented.

4.2.   LASER BEAM PROPAGATION IN ATMOSPHERIC TURBULENCE

Background[1,2,3,4,5]

When a laser beam traverses a distance in the atmosphere, its ideal phase characteristics experience small perturbations which alter and redirect the energy in the beam. The resulting intensity fluctuations are called scintillations and have been observed by all of us in looking at twinkling stars. The source of these perturbations is a random index of refraction field. The source of this field is related through the density almost exclusively to temperature fluctuations. Pressure variations (P) are very small and are rapidly dispersed. One can therefore show that the change in the index of refraction with temperature (T) in the atmosphere (using an isobaric assumption) is given by

$$\Delta n(r) = -79 \times 10^{-6} \frac{P}{T^2} \Delta T(r) \ . \tag{1}$$

It is generally assumed that the atmosphere is at least locally homogeneous and isotropic, though this is often not true. To help diminish the problems associated with this assumption, atmospheric scientists often studied structure functions. Defined as

$$D_n(r_1, r_2) = \langle \{ [n(r_1) - \langle n(r_1) \rangle] \tag{2}$$

$$- [n(r_2) - \langle n(r_2) \rangle] \}^2 \rangle \ ,$$

where the brackets denote ensemble average, this function has been found to be less sensitive in form to the conditions of local homogeneity and isotropy. Assuming homogeneous and isotropic turbulence, the temperature field has been shown experimentally and theoretically for sufficiently small spacings (r) to have the form

$$D_T(r) = \langle [\Delta T(p) - \Delta T(r+p)]^2 \rangle = C_T^2 r^{2/3}. \tag{3}$$

Using high speed temperature sensitive instruments, one can calculate the constant C_T^6. Through Eq. (1) a similar spatial dependence of the index of refraction can be obtained and hence a determination of C_n^2 made. We find

$$C_n^2 = \left(\frac{79P}{T^2} 10^{-6} \right)^2 C_T^2 . \tag{4}$$

C_n^2 is frequently called the atmospheric structure "constant," although it is seldom very constant. It has come to typify in one all encompassing term the nature or strength of the atmospheric turbulence. Its value ranges from 10^{-17} $m^{-2/3}$ or smaller for very weak turbulence to 10^{-13} $m^{-2/3}$ or larger for very strong turbulence. Actually, the nature of atmospheric turbulence is much too complicated to be described very well by this one parameter. Notably, scale sizes are very important in the description of naturally occurring turbulence.

Temperature fluctuations are introduced into the atmosphere by large scale phenomena such as heating of the earth's surface. These disturbances are broken up and mixed by the wind until temperature fluctuations of all scale sizes exist. Wind fluctuations control the temperature variations. Hence it is instructive to discuss the characteristics of the atmospheric wind field.

This field obtains energy from large scales such as wind shear or convection from solar heating of the ground. Therefore, the turbulence energy must be introduced by scale sizes larger than some minimum value (L_o) called the outer scale of turbulence. (Wave number $K_o = 2\pi/L_o$ in Fig. 1.*) For $K < K_o$, the form of the power spectrum is not known in general owing to its dependence on local conditions and surface terrain. In this region the turbulence is most likely not homogeneous and isotropic. Typical sizes for L_o vary from a number like the height

---

*   Actually, Fig. 1 shows the power spectrum of the index of refraction fluctuations, but the form of the curve is equivalent to the velocity field power spectrum as well.

above ground to 100 meters or more for the upper atmosphere though stratification can alter this.   In Fig. 1,
the inclusion of a finite outer scale causes the power
spectrum to remain finite as $K \to 0$.

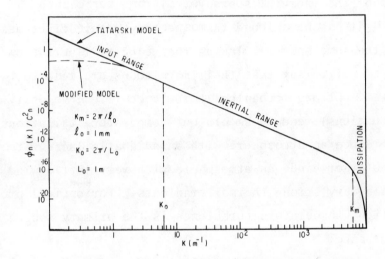

*Fig. 1.   Three-dimensional spectrum of the refractive
index fluctuations (Ref. 4).*

Under the assumptions that energy is input at the
small wave numbers and dissipated at large wave number,
and that for these scale sizes of turbulence the Reynolds
number is much greater than unity, and that the scale
sizes are small enough so that buoyancy forces are negligible, Kolmogorov originally proposed a turbulence model
that predicted a $K^{-11/3}$ spectrum in the inertial subrange
where the scale sizes are smaller than L_O, but larger
than ℓ_O; this has been experimentally verfied. ℓ_O is an
inner scale length which marks the turbulence scale sizes
for which viscous dissipation converts the energy in the

turbulence into heat. Typically it is on the order of 1 mm near the ground to a few millimeters at altitude. In this region of the turbulence spectrum, the form is again not well known. However, it is clear that for $K > K_m = 5.92/\ell_o$, the slope of the spectrum is steeper than the slope of the inertial subrange.

It has been found that the temperature fluctuations obey the same spectral law as the velocity fluctuations. That is not to say that their magnitudes are related, however. Strong mechanical turbulence (i.e., velocity fluctuations) tend to smooth out temperature variations and produce an atmosphere with an adiabatic lapse rate. On the other hand, an atmosphere with very little wind can sustain very strong thermal gradients. For optical pro-pagation, temperature turbulence is the primary source of disturbance.

Tatarski[1] used the following form for the power spectrum of the refractive index:

$$\Phi_n(K) = 0.033\ C_n^2\ K^{-11/3}\ \exp(-K^2/K_m^2). \qquad (5)$$

This spectrum is singular at $K = 0$ and therefore does not possess a covariance function. This difficulty can be circumvented by use of a Von Karman spectrum of the form[4]

$$\Phi_n(K) = \frac{0.033\ C_n^2\ \exp(-K^2/K_m^2)}{[K^2 + (L_o/2\pi)^{-2}]^{11/6}} \qquad (6)$$

that artificially imposes a well behaved dependence for $K \to 0$.

In Fig. 2 some experimental results are presented
to show[7] the simultaneous behavior of the measurement of
optical intensity scintillation and C_n^2. Plotted on the
ordinate is the variance of the log amplitude $\sigma_\chi^2 =$
$\langle (\chi - \langle \chi \rangle)^2 \rangle$, where $\chi = ln(A/A_o)$, A_o and A being
the unperturbed and perturbed field amplitudes, respec-
tively (note $I \sim A^2$, where I is the field irradiance).
The theoretical log amplitude variance prediction for a
spherical wave source in turbulence is

$$\sigma_\chi^2 = 0.124 \; C_n^2 \; Z^{11/6} \; k^{7/6}$$

where $k = 2\pi/\lambda$, λ is the optical wavelength, and Z is
the range to the observation plane. These results show
the good agreement between macroscopic measurements of
turbulence and simultaneous optical effects. Note the
increased strength of both processes during daylight hours,
the very low values at sunrise and sunset and the night-
time variability. The two simultaneous optical path measurements also show the frequently referred to phenomenon
of saturation of scintillation[8,9,10,11]; during daylight
hours, the variance of the log irradiance of the 1000 m
path is actually lower than the same quantity measured in
the 490 m path. This behavior has frequently been
observed and is really only understood in principle to be
a multi-scattering phenomenon.

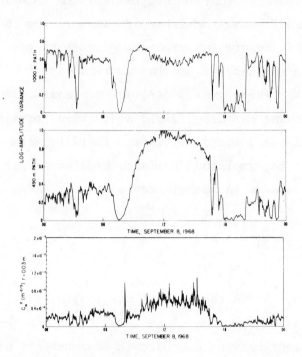

*Fig. 2.   Simultaneous amplitude scintillation and
          turbulence structure constant data (Ref. 7).*

Propagation Of Beam Waves In A Turbulent Atmosphere

Historically one finds that much of the original
experimental and theoretical work has been directed at
studying the propagation effects of plane and spherical
wave sources in a turbulent medium. In recent years there
has been considerable interest in extending the earlier
theories to treat the propagation of beam waves in turbulence. The theoretical work has been extensive[12-24] and
presents many interesting questions which need to be tested
by the experimentalist. Unfortunately, experimental results on beam wave propagation have been slow in

developing,[22-27] owing mainly to the difficulties associated with good quality large laser optics and related
instrumentation. I confine my remaining discussion of
atmospheric turbulence effects to those results which
specifically apply to the propagation of beam waves. (A
beam wave may be defined as any transmission configuration
which does not fall in the spherical wave or plane wave
propagation case. Stated slightly differently, it may be
defined as a propagation arrangement in which the transmitted beam immerges from optics which have finite size).

   Consider an experimental arrangement (Fig. 3) in
which a beam wave is transmitted through atmospheric turbulence to a target where it is observed. The transmitter
characteristics are specified by the output beam diameter
(D), the wavelength (λ), and the focal length (F). The
intervening turbulence is specified by the structure constant (C_n^2), and the outer and inner scale sizes. If
$L_o > D$, then there must be turbulence scale sizes that are
larger than the beam diameter at all points along the beam
path. These "turbules" act as weak lenses which deflect
the beam as a whole in a random way leaving the shape of
the beam unaltered. This is called beam wander. Scale

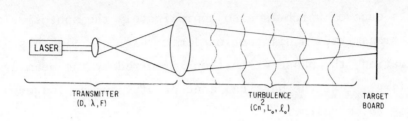

Fig. 3. Usual propagation configuration.

sizes smaller than the diameter of the beam diffract and refract the beam and generally smear-out its energy distribution profile, an effect referred to as beam breathing and scintillation. Depending on the characteristics of the turbulence and the transmitter, these two mechanisms share with some proportion in producing the total "average long term" distortion of the beam. Kerr[23] has observed that under moderate strengths of turbulence, the focal plane distribution retains its diffraction limited beam size but moves randomly mainly under the influence of the large turbulence scale sizes (Fig. 4). He has observed large scintillation effects, however, at points well removed from the central spot of the beam. The reduction in scintillation of the central spot is predicted in one beam wave theory,[12] but the same theory apparently fails to adequately account for the beam wander effects.[23] This theory also predicts a severe sensitivity of scintillation of focus adjustments, an effect which Kerr found to be true (Fig. 5). Misadjustments in focus resulted in a beam which scintillated strongly in the form of many time evolving intensity blobs each of which is approximately the size of the transmitter's diffraction limit. In the presence of strong turbulence, the beam breaks up into a proliferation of many spots each of which is also approximately the spot size of the transmitter's diffraction limit (Fig. 6). In this situation, the phase distortions incurred by the beam are so large, that the physical concept of focus no longer seems to be valid.

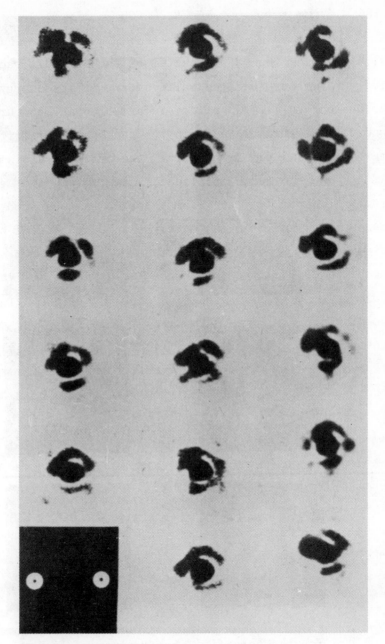

Fig. 4. *Characteristic received beam for a focused, near-field transmitter in moderate turbulence. The duration of each frame was 4 ms; the time between adjacent frames was 21 ms. The frame sequence is downward in each column, and the scale marks represent 2.5 cm. $\lambda = 4880\text{Å}$, $L = 1.4$ km, $D_T = 15$ cm, $\alpha_1 L = 0.09$ (Ref. 23).*

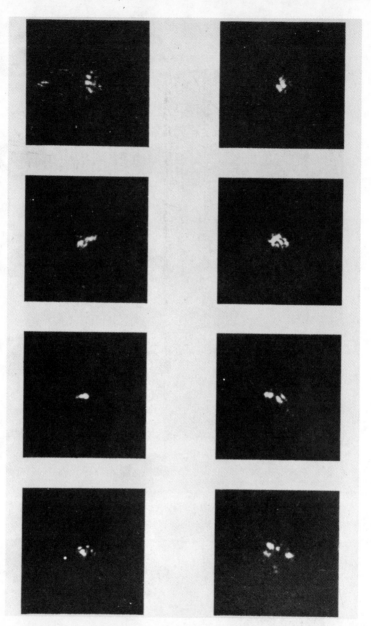

Fig. 5. Received beam vs transmitter focal adjustment for the near-field transmitter of Fig. 4 in moderate turbulence. Successive frames downward represent axial focal adjustments of 50 μm compared to an effective focal length of 120 cm. Precise focus is illustrated in the third frame. Individual patches have the same nominal size as the central spot in Fig. 4 (Ref. 23).

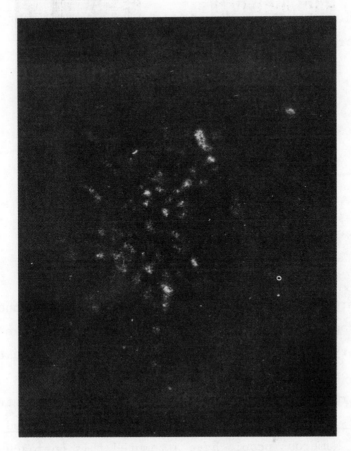

Fig. 6.   *Received beam for the focused, near-field
transmitter of Fig. 4 in strong turbulence.
Individual patches have the same nominal size
as the central spot in Fig. 4 (Ref. 23).*

A problem closely related to the propagation configuration of Fig. 3 is shown in Fig. 7. If one observes
the image plane characteristics of the point source, he
will find almost exactly the same characteristic dependences as Kerr found for the beam wave projected through

the turbulence. This is no accident, and it is related to
the reciprocity of the linear turbulence operator.

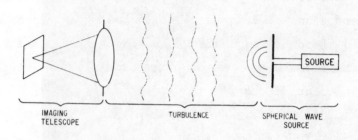

IMAGING
TELESCOPE   TURBULENCE   SPHERICAL WAVE
                                                      SOURCE

Fig. 7. Reciprocal propagation configuration.

For example, beam wander is clearly a major concern
in the propagation of beam waves, for there exists the
possibility that this phenomenon can be removed by fast
tracking optical systems. Because the beam wander is
mainly a result of large turbulence scale sizes, geometrical optics approaches to the problem should yield good
results. Numerous people have attempted this approach
making a special treatment of turbulence scale sizes which
are larger than (or smaller) than the beam size.[24,26]
Hull et al.,[24] using such an approach obtained the following expression for the angular beam wander (along one axis)

$$<\alpha^2> \ = \ \frac{3}{4} LD^{-1/3} \ C_n^{\ 2} \left\{ 1.46 - \frac{8}{9} \ (D/L_o)^{1/3} \right\}. \quad (7)$$

Considering the reciprocal problem (Fig. 7), several other people have analyzed the nature of the focal plane
image dancing.[3,15,16,20,27] Fried,[27] for instance, used an
approach that decomposed the turbulence distorted phase

profile at the collecting aperture into a series of polynomials. He then defined the angle of arrival as the angle
normal to the best fit linear plane surface through the
phase aberrations. Hiedbreder,[16] also using an extremum
approach defined the angle formed in the direction of maximum instantaneous power as the beam wander. Both workers
arrived at identical results for image dancing.[20]

In the limit $L_o \to \infty$, they obtained (for spherical
waves)

$$\langle \alpha^2 \rangle \;=\; (2.91)(3/8)(1.026)LD^{-1/3} C_n^2 \tag{8}$$

which differs from Eq. (7) by about 1%. The thrust of the
image dancing analysis can be easily visualized in the following argument originally proposed by Hufnagel.[19] Consider an arbitrary phase distribution across an aperture of
diameter D. The phase difference between opposite points
on the edge of the aperture is $[\phi(D/2,0) - \phi(-D/2,0)]$ so
that the angular tilt is just

$$\alpha \;=\; [\phi(D/2,0) - \phi(-D/2,0)]/kD \tag{9}$$

where $k = 2\pi/\lambda$. Assuming a zero mean for α, one gets
for the variance

$$\langle \alpha^2 \rangle \;=\; D_s(D)/k^2 D^2 \tag{10}$$

where $D_s(\cdot)$ is the phase structure function. For a spherical wave, and $L_o \to \infty$, and $D > \sqrt{\lambda L}$

$$\langle \alpha^2 \rangle \;=\; (2.91)\,(3/8)LD^{-1/3}\,C_n^{\,2} \tag{11}$$

which is quite similar to Eq. (8). Inclusion of outer scale effects produces

$$\langle \alpha^2 \rangle \;=\; (2.91)\,(3/8)LD^{-1/3}\,C_n^{\,2}\,[1-0.67(D/\mathcal{L}_o)^{1/3}] \tag{12}$$

where $\mathcal{L}_o = L_o/2\pi$. The existence of a finite outer scale tends to decrease the strength of the beam wander.[14]

Beam wander has been measured by a few researchers under varying conditions of transmitter configuration and turbulence strengths.[22,23,24,26] Some of the most interesting work was performed by Dowling et al. at Naval Research Laboratories (NRL), where they simultaneously measured through common optics the far field irradiance characteristics of laser radiation of two very different wavelengths (.6328 μm and 10.6 μm). Their results show, among other things, that beam wander is to a very high degree independent of wavelength (Fig. 8) as the theory predicts and a reasonably accurate function of $LC_n^{\,2}$ (Fig. 9). Maximum values of $\langle \alpha^2 \rangle$ exceeded 1.6×10^{-8} μrad² at times of strong turbulence.

The developments leading to Eqs. (7), (8), (11), and (12) stress the importance of the phase structure function. To include amplitude effects, the wave structure function, defined as the sum of the phase and log amplitude structure functions, should be used instead. However, for many situations of interest, the effects of phase aberrations strongly outweigh the comparable amplitude effects

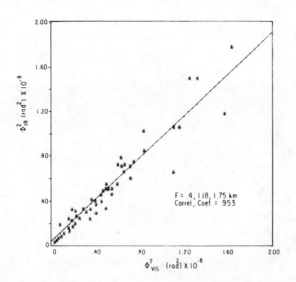

*Fig. 8.   Experimental beam wander data for a visible
            and an infrared beam (Ref. 22).*

and can be shown to dominate the far field distributions.
Nonetheless, it should be kept in mind that these developments have assumed small amplitude disturbances.   In any
event amplitude effects should never produce more than a
factor of two effects in the calculations.

The reciprocity of beam wander (Fig. 3) and image
dancing (Fig. 7) is only part of a very useful *reciprocity
theorem*.   It may be stated as follows.[29]   Consider a single realization of the random index of refraction field
between two points in space ($\underline{p}_1$ and $\underline{p}_2$).   The field at
point $\underline{p}_1$ due to a unit amplitude spherical wave source at
point $\underline{p}_2$ is exactly the same as the field at $\underline{p}_2$ due to a
unit amplitude spherical wave source at point $\underline{p}_1$.   Any
linear refractive element (say, for example, a lens) may
be placed between $\underline{p}_1$ and $\underline{p}_2$, and the reciprocity theorem
is still valid.

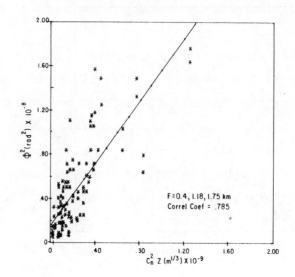

Fig. 9. *Experimental beam wander as a function of*
        $C_n{}^2 Z$ *(Ref. 22).*

        There are a number of important implications of
this result. First, one can show that if the instantaneous
phase and amplitude distribution can be measured in the
transmitting aperture for point source located at the
receiver plane, then by transmitting a beam whose amplitude and phase is exactly conjugate to this, the far field
irradiance distribution is only limited by the diffraction
aspects of the telescope. This is to say, all the dele-
terious effects of the intervening turbulence can be
eliminated. Of course, it is no simple feat to either
instantaneously measure the amplitude and phase of the
point source accurately, or to quickly and precisely generate a beam with the conjugate field distribution. However, there does exist the possibility of rapidly sensing
(through heterodyne detection, for instance) an effective
wavefront tilt for the spherical wave. Transmitting a
beam with the conjugate tilt (fast tracking telescopes do

this) can eliminate the beam wander component of the phase distortion.

Another consequence of the point to point reciprocity theorem is that even if a refractive lens (or a whole telescope, for that matter) is inserted between the two point sources, the reciprocity of the field is still valid. Tracking wavefront tilt only varies the position in the focal plane of the lens where the exact field reciprocity exists. Thus, rather than measure the actual phase front of the point source, one need simply sense the position of the focal plane spot (energy centroid, peak power, etc.) in order to generate corrective signal for wavefront tilt compensation.

Actually, there is a qualification to the above results that I failed to mention. For this method of wavefront tilt compensation to be valid, the nature of the turbulence and the propagation phenomenon must be such that the beam spot size and the required angular wander compensation be small compared to the isoplanatic patch size. To put it another way, suppose a single realization of the turbulence is frozen in time. Suppose we transmit two identical beams through the same telescope, to two very close positions in the receiver plane. If the two irradiance patterns are exactly alike (this, of course, needs some qualifications), aside from the projected lateral displacement, then the two images are well within the isoplanatic patch size, and the technique of using focal plane spot displacement to sense wavefront tilt is valid. Incidentally, this condition is usually satisfied for beams focused in the near field of the transmitter.

Under these conditions, one can also show that the
irradiance pattern of a point source obtained in the focal
plane of the telescope when it is used as a receiving
optic and the irradiance pattern obtained in the focal
plane for a beam projected from the telescope through the
turbulence will, instantaneously, be exactly the same. In
addition, the qualification regarding the beam size and
the isoplanatic patch size can be totally removed if one
considers instead statistical quantities, such as, for
instance, the long time average smear size of the beam.

Using this theorem, Lutomirski and Yura[13,31] (L&Y)
have developed an elegant propagation theory which seems
to coalesce nicely with the few recorded experimental
observations of beam wave propagation which are available
for detailed comparison. Hufnagel and Stanley,[19] Fried,[18]
and Mooreland and Collins[17] developed a similar line of
analysis for the case of an imaging receiver. By the
reciprocity theorem, they are now known to be the same.
L&Y show that the irradiance at a point $\vec{p}$ in the receiver
plane is given by[13]

$$I(\vec{p}) = \left(\frac{k}{2\pi Z}\right)^2 \iint \exp\{ik(s_1 - s_2)\}$$

(13)

$$\times \exp\{\psi(\vec{r}_1) + \psi^*(\vec{r}_2)\} U_A^*(\vec{r}_2)\, d\vec{r}_1^{\,2} d\vec{r}_2^{\,2},$$

where $U_A(\vec{r})$ is the transmitted aperture distribution;
s_1, s_2 are the geometric distances between points $\vec{p}$ and
the points $\vec{r}_1$ and $\vec{r}_2$ in the aperture, respectively; and

$\Psi(\vec{r}_1)$ and $\Psi(\vec{r}_2)$ are the perturbations in the field at $\vec{p}$ due to unit spherical waves emitted at $\vec{r}_1$ and $\vec{r}_2$.

Performing an ensemble average, or as is done in practice averaging over a time long compared to all the beam wander and beam scintillation frequencies of interest, one gets

$$<I(\vec{p})>_{LT} = \left(\frac{k}{2\pi Z}\right)^2 \iint \exp[ik(s_1-s_1)] M_s^{LT}(\vec{r}_1, \vec{r}_2, Z)$$

$$\times \ U(\vec{r}_1) U^*(\vec{r}_1) d^2\vec{r}_1 d^2\vec{r}_2,$$

(14)

where M_s^{LT} is the "long time" mutual coherence function of a point source located at the receiver plane and measured at the transmitter plane. One can readily show that if $\Psi(r_1) = \chi + iS$, where $\chi = ln(A/A_o)$ (A_o being the unperturbed amplitude of the field, and A the perturbed amplitude) and where S is the perturbation to the phase, then assuming that the random quantities are gaussian random variables,

$$M_s^{LT}(\rho, z) = <\exp[\Psi(\vec{r}_1) \ \Psi^*(\vec{r}_2)]>$$

$$= \exp\{-D(p)/2\},$$

(15)

where $|\vec{r}_1 - \vec{r}_2| = p$ and where $D(p)$ is the wave structure function given by

$$D(p) = D\chi(p) + D_S(p).$$

(16)

Homogeneous and isotropic turbulence has been assumed. In
terms of the covariance function (instead of structure
functions)

$$D(\rho) = 2[B(0) - B(\rho)], \tag{17}$$

$B(0)$ is a constant and is equal to the sum variances of
the log amplitude fluctuations and the phase fluctuations.
$B(\rho)$ is the covariance function which can assume many
forms, but in general has the property that as $\rho \to \infty$,
$B(\rho) = 0$. Thus a typical form for the mutual coherence
function in Eq. (14) might be like the function shown in
Fig. 10. L&Y show that the asymptotic limit is given by

$$B(0) = 2Z/Z_c, \tag{18}$$

where

$$Z_c = [2\pi^2 k^2 \int_0^\infty \Phi_n(K) K\, K]^{-1} . \tag{19}$$

For $\ell_o \ll L_o$, (19) can be approximated by

$$Z_c \approx (0.4 k^2 C_n^2 L_o^{5/3})^{-1} \tag{20}$$

Notice that in the limit of infinitely large L_o [as implied
by the power spectrum of Eq. (5)], $Z_c = 0$. This is a
reflection of implication that there is, in this limit, an
infinite amount of energy in the turbulence spectrum,
which of course is not true. Nonetheless, if one holds

all else constant, then by increasing the outer scale size
the total energy in the turbulence spectrum grows, and
hence more severe optical effects occur. Thus, it is
valid to conclude that when Eq. (5) can be used to calculate optical quantities, the results generally form an
upper limit estimate of the effects. This is illustrated
in the comments that follow. Z_c has units of length, and
may be thought of as designating a propagation distance
for which the mean field of a spherical wave is reduced by
e^{-1} from its vacuum value.

For homogeneous and isotropic turbulence, Eq. (14)
can be written in the paraxial approximation as

$$<I(\vec{p})> \ = \ \left(\frac{k}{2\pi Z}\right)^2 \iint d^2\vec{\rho}\ M_s^{LT}(\vec{\rho},z) \exp[-(ik/z)\vec{\rho}\cdot\vec{p}]$$

$$\times \iint U(\vec{r}+\vec{p}/2)U^*(\vec{r}-\vec{p}/2)$$

$$\times \ \exp[(ik/z)\vec{\rho}\cdot\vec{r}]d^2\vec{r}\ , \qquad\qquad (21)$$

where the second double integral can be identified as the
Modulation Transfer Function of the transmitter. This
function varies in shape dependence on the nature of the
telescope and radiation source, but generally might have
a shape as shown in Fig. 10 (bottom curve). As the diameter of the transmitted beam is increased, or the wavelength of the radiation shortened, the cut-off frequency
grows larger indicating an increase in the resolution of
the telescope (and conversely, indicating a decrease in
the transmitted diffraction limited spot size).

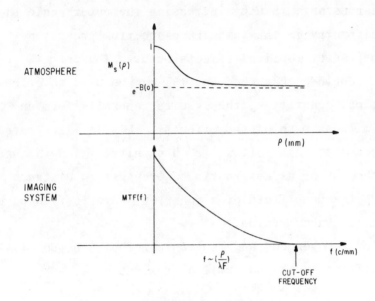

*Fig. 10. Typical modulation transfer functions for the
atmosphere, and for a telescope.*

Consequently, Eq. (21) can be interpreted as
stating that the MTF of the total system (atmosphere and
telescope) is the product of the.MTF of the atmosphere and
the MTF of the telescope. The irradiance distribution
(point spread function) is just the Fourier transform of
the total system MTF.

Clearly, if $M_s^{LT}(\vec{\rho}) = 1$, (for all $\vec{\rho}$), the system
is diffraction limited, the integral argument being dominated by the MTF of the telescope. In fact, if $\exp[-B(0)]$
is greater than say e^{-1}, the effects of turbulence on the
optical transmission characteristics are very slight. If,
however, $\exp[-B(0)] \ll e^{-1}$, the atmosphere has a strong
effect on the beam. The degree to which the effect is
severe depends critically on the width of $M_s^{LT}(\rho)$. L&Y
arbitrarily define a (long term) "coherence diameter" as
being that value of $\rho = \rho_o$ for which $M_s^{LT}(\rho_o^{LT}) = e^{-1}$.

In order to be able to do this, one must require of the propagation range being considered that $M_s(\ell_o, Z) \simeq 1$ and $M_s(L_o, Z) \ll 1$ which implies that

$$Z_c \ll Z \ll Z_i, \tag{22}$$

where $Z_i = Z_c(L_o/\ell_o)^{5/3}$. In this region, one can write approximately that

$$M_s^{LT}(\rho, z) = \exp[-1.4(Z/Z_c)(\rho/\not{E}_o)^{5/3}$$

$$\times \ (1-0.71 \ (\rho/\not{E}_o)^{1/3})] \tag{23}$$

and

$$\rho_o^{LT}(L_o) \simeq \rho_o^{LT}(\infty)(1 + 0.426[\rho_o^{LT}(\infty)/\not{E}_o]^{1/3}), \tag{24}$$

where $\rho_o(\infty) = (0.545 \ ZC_n^2 k^2)^{-3/5}$ is the coherence diameter obtained by assuming an infinitely large outer scale (i.e., using Eq. (5) for the power spectrum).

If $Z \gg Z_i$, then $M_s^{LT}(\ell_o, Z) \ll 1$ and the focal plane irradiance distribution is very broad. The $M_s^{LT}(\rho)$ is found there to depend most strongly on the inner scale characteristics:

$$M_s^{LT}(\rho) = \exp[0.8(Z/Z_i)(\rho/\ell_o)^2]. \tag{25}$$

For this case,

$$\rho_o = [0.76 \, C_n^2 \, Z^{1/2} \, \ell_o^{-1/6} \, k]^{-1} \ll \ell_o. \qquad (26)$$

One can then interpret the preceding results as follows. Turbulence converts a coherent radiator of diameter D into a partially coherent radiator of diameter ρ_o^{LT}. The size of ρ_o^{LT} is determined solely by the Mutual Coherence Function of a spherical wave source located at the receiver and measured in the transmitter plane. Incidentally, to be more precise, in the range where $Z_c \le Z \le Z_i$, and $L_o \to \infty$, ρ_o is given by the following weighted integral.

$$\rho_o^{LT} \simeq \left[1.45 k^2 \int_{Z_1}^{Z_2} C_n^2(Z') \left[\frac{Z_2 - Z'}{Z_2 - Z_1} \right]^{5/3} dZ' \right]^{-3/5}. \qquad (27)$$

This implies that the turbulence *near the transmitter* (Z_1) is weighted most heavily as affecting the beam propagation characteristics. Thus, for instance, if atmospheric turbulence can be assumed to decrease with altitude, then ground based illuminators of airborne receivers are degraded more seriously than equivalent airborne illuminators of ground based receivers.

The relative size of ρ_o^{LT} to D has been found to correlate well with observations made by Kerr. The following conclusions apply to a beam focused in the near field of the transmitting aperture. Namely, when $\rho_o^{LT} \gg D$, no turbulence effects of any degree are significant. For $\rho_o^{LT} \approx D$, beam wander is found to be the predominant propagation effect, with very little instantaneous beam breathing or scintillation. For $\rho_o^{LT} \le D$, beam wander is still a major effect, but now beam breathing is becoming

a competing process, though still not dominant.   If
ρ_O^{LT} << D, scintillation, and beam spreading are the
dominant effects.

Amplitude scintillation effects are small when Z is
in the near field of the ρ_O^{LT} or D, whichever is smaller,
i.e., $Z \leq k \rho_O^{LT^2}$.   (This condition coincides nicely with
the requirement that the amplitude scintillation of a
spherical wave remain small).   For $Z > k\rho_O^{LT^2}$, where
ρ_O << D the beam breaks up into a proliferation of individual patches of spots, each approximately the diffraction
spot size of the transmitting aperture.   Focusing in this
case ceases to have a well defined meaning.

One implication of the preceding which is important
is that when $Z \leq Z_c$, substantial improvement in far field
irradiance can be achieved by using increasingly larger
transmitting optics (see Ref. 16).   This conclusion however, does not follow if the power spectrum of Eq. (5) is
used.   In that case, the MCF is found to be given by

$$M_s(\rho) = \exp[-(2.91)(3/8)k^2 C_n^2 Z \rho^{5/3}] \tag{28}$$

which rapidly tends to an asymptotic value of zero for
large ρ, (i.e., $Z_c \to 0$ as $L_o \to 0$ as noted before).
Recalling the form of the calculation of the irradiance
distribution, the quantity of interest is the product of
the atmospheric and telescopic MCF's.   If the aperture of
the transmitter is made sufficiently large, its MCF becomes
wider than the atmospheric MCF (Fig. 10), so that the integral in Eq. (21) is determined solely from the form of the
latter MCF.   When Eq. (28) is used for the form of the
atmospheric MCF, this implies that the maximum far field

irradiance achievable with increasingly larger transmitting optics is limited.   (See Fig. 11 from Ref. 16).
With the inclusion of outer scale effects, and the assumption that $2Z/Z_c \lesssim 1$, the correct form of the atmospheric
MCF shows an asymptotic limiting values as $\rho \to \infty$ of
$\exp(-2Z/Z_c)$.   The area under this curve grows without
limit (conceptually) so that by making the MCF of the telescope broader $(D \to \infty)$, the far field irradiance can be continually (and substantially) improved.   (See Fig. 11).   For
values of $Z/Z_c \gg 1$, the differences in the shapes of the
atmospheric MCF's became less significant, with the result
that for all practical purposes the maximum irradiance in
the far field <u>does</u> saturate with increasing transmitting
aperture diameter.

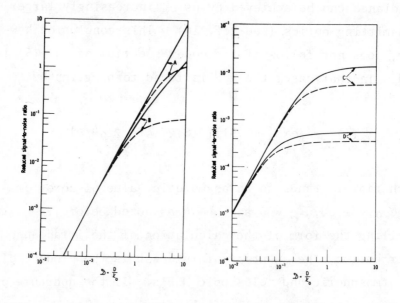

*Fig. 11.   Reduced S/N ratios of far field irradiance as
          functions of collector diameter (in units of t_o).
          Curves A, B, C and D correspond to z/z_c = 0.1,
          1.0, 10 and 100 respectively.*

Recently Yura[15] has developed a similar formalism
to describe "short-time" propagation effects. These effects only include the average instantaneous beam characteristics, beam wander being filtered out of the long time
atmospheric MCF. Yura's results follow from the development of the short time MCF (due to Fried[18]) and really
only apply when scintillation effects are small. One gets
that

$$M_s^{ST}(\rho) = \exp\left\{-\left(\frac{\rho}{\rho_o^{LT}}\right)^{5/3}\left[1-0.62(\rho/D)^{1/3}\right]\right\}, \quad (29)$$

where this is valid when $\rho \gg (\lambda Z)^{1/2}$, $L_o = \infty$ (and consequently for $Z_c \lesssim Z \lesssim Z_i$). Proceeding as before, one can
define an approximate short time lateral coherence diameter
as

$$\rho_o^{ST} = \rho_o^{LT}\left[1 + 0.37 (\rho_o^{LT}/D)^{1/3}\right]. \quad (30)$$

The implications are that if one can track out (or in some
other manner remove) the beam wander, the effective atmospheric MCF is broadened, with a subsequent increase in
the effective coherence diameter of the radiator. One
might then alter the preceding interpretation of the experimental results by replacing everything that was said
about ρ_o^{LT} by ρ_o^{ST}. The fact of the matter is, however,
that these parameters do not differ greatly anyway, so
that the thrust of the argument is still very much the
same.

Yura[30] also shows that one can obtain an approximate estimate for the size of the irradiance distribution (defined to the e^{-1} point) as

$$p_1^2 = p_o^2 + p_T^2 , \qquad (31)$$

where

$$p_o = \frac{2Z}{kD}$$

and

$$p_T = \frac{2Z}{kp_o^{LT}} \quad \text{or} \quad \frac{2Z}{kp_o^{ST}}$$

depending on the specific problem of interest. One can then make an argument for the approximate independence of the beam wander and beam spreading processes and assert that the two random effects can be r.m.s.'ed as

$$\langle \alpha^2 \rangle = (p_{LT}^2 - p_{ST}^2)/Z^2 \qquad (32)$$

which can be compared with the work described earlier for beam wander. The agreement in functional dependence is exact, but they differ in magnitude by about 20%, the latter angular variance being smaller. This is probably a reflection of the inappropriateness of the r.m.s. assumption, though this has not been shown.

In Eq. (29), it is clear that as $D \to \infty$, the long time and short time effects cease to be different.

Physically this corresponds to situations where the transmitting aperture size is larger than almost all the turbulence scale sizes of interest. Spatial averaging of the
turbulence over the width of the beam only produces beam
spreading, beam wander becoming a secondary effect. In
view of this observation and with the possibility of tracking out beam wander, the curves in Fig. 11 now appear as
shown in Fig. 12. Removing beam wander can produce a system with an optimum far field irradiance that is larger
than the large aperture limiting value. Subsequent increase
in transmitting aperture size actually leads to a decrease
in system performance (though very slowly). The two upper
curves utilize the two different beam wander approaches,
Yura's approach being the lower of the two. The lowest
curve not exceeding the asymptotic value is the same as
the curves shown in Fig. 11 with $L_O \to \infty$.

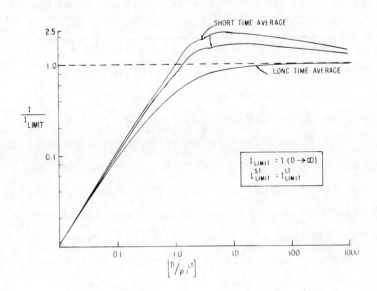

Fig. 12.　Average focal plane maximum irradiance dependence
on transmitter aperture size, for long term and
short term averages.

I have not mentioned wavelength dependence in this
problem. Clearly beam wander is a wavelength independent
phenomenon; however, beam spreading is not, and it does
exhibit a weak theoretical wavelength dependence. To
illustrate the dependence, consider two systems. Both systems are operating with the same total output power, transmitter diameter, focal length setting and wavelength of
radiation. The first system *does not* have the ability to
track beam wander whereas the second system does, and this
is their only difference. Pose the following problem: if
one is at liberty to alter the wavelength of the source
radiation, what transmitting aperture size produces the
same far field irradiance maxima? The results for the
first system are shown in Fig. 13. In the absence of turbulence, the dashed line indicates the appropriate system
and therefore the ideal aperture. With turbulence, however, one finds that he needs apertures which are slightly
larger than the ideal limit, indicating that turbulence is
affecting the shorter wavelengths more severely. In
addition, there is a limiting wavelength, below which no
finite aperture can achieve the equivalent irradiance
(again I have used the case where $Z >> Z_c$).

When beam wander is removed, one observes a similar
behavior shown in Fig. 14. Note that since wander has
been removed, these curves represent an effectively higher
maximum irradiance, and yet, the optimum wavelength is
actually less than for the long time average case. The
explanation for this is related to the fact that beam
wander is not wavelength dependent. Consequently, the
effect of a particular value of beam wander on the far
field irradiance is proportionally larger for the shorter

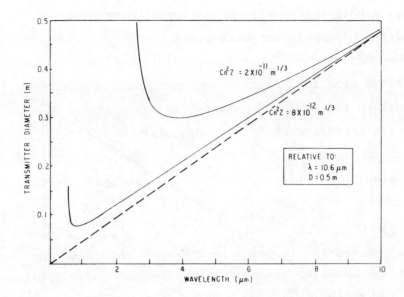

Fig. 13. *Equivalent transmitting systems that produce constant focal plane maximum intensity for different strengths of turbulence (long term average).*

wavelength system. Of course, all of these conclusions assume that the observation plane is in the near field of the spherical wave lateral coherence diameter in order to assure small amplitude scintillation effects.

I might point out that this curve is not asymptotic at this apparent value of wavelength. Actually, with increasing transmitter diameter, the corresponding system equivalent wavelength begins to increase again, eventually asymptoting a wavelength that is larger than the limiting wavelength in Fig. 13. This is to be expected, since the curves in Fig. 14 correspond to a higher system equivalent irradiance than the ones in Fig. 13. The limiting intensity as $D \to \infty$ can be easily shown to vary as $\lambda^{2/5}$, and therefore a longer wavelength system is needed in order to

achieve the proportionally higher irradiance value
obtained by tracking out beam wander.

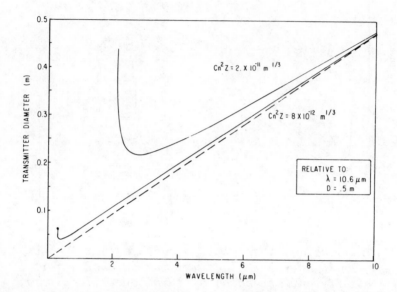

Fig. 14.   *Equivalent transmitting systems that produce*
constant focal plane maximum intensity for
different strengths of turbulence (long term
average).

Thus, even though there is only a weak dependence
on the radiation wavelength, its inclusion in the turbulence problem can in some situations strongly alter the
final system design considerations.

4.3. LASER BEAM PROPAGATION IN AN ABSORBING MEDIUM

Background

The propagation of laser beams in turbulence is a
linear process in that the medium is not perturbed by the
presence of the radiation. Strictly speaking, this is only
true for very low power beams. As the energy is increased,
absorption of the radiation begins to induce temperature
changes in the medium, which, in turn, result in density,
and therefore index of refraction changes. These then
alter the optical characteristics of the medium. The process is nonlinear, in that the beam irradiance distribution
induces index of refraction changes in the medium which in
turn alters the beam irradiance characteristics, which
alters the refractive index changes, ..., etc.

In the past, one basic problem has received a great
deal of attention in the open literature.[32-42] Specifically, the following assumptions were usually made with
regard to the thermal blooming problem: 1) the high energy beam has an unperturbed irradiance profile that is
gaussian shape; 2) the medium through which the beam passes
is flowing at a constant velocity that is much less than
the speed of sound and is free of any turbulence (i.e.,
laminar flow); 3) the beam is assumed to have been "on" for
a time long enough to establish a steady state irradiance
distribution; 4) the wavelength of the radiation is 10.6
μm; and finally, it has been assumed that 5) the energy
thermalization process produces an instantaneous heating
of the medium. In addition, using assumption 2), it can

be shown that the hydrodynamic processes of interest are
essentially isobaric, and therefore an instantaneous temperature change in the medium causes an instantaneous density change and therefore refractive index change.

In this section, I discuss the nature of the results
obtained for the basic thermal blooming problem described
by the assumptions above. In addition, some recent work on
related subjects will also be presented. The discussion
begins with a brief review of the basic thermal blooming
problem.

Basic Problem Considerations

With the five assumptions specified above, the
thermo-optical process is conceptually easy to visualize.
Figure 15 is a simplified description of what is known as
pure blooming. Holding assumption 2) in abeyance for the
moment, let us assume that the air is stationary, so that
at $t = 0$ second, the temperature, density, and index of
refraction profile are constant across the beam. When the
beam has been turned on, some of the radiation energy is
absorbed and then released in the form of heat in the gas;
the temperature in the vicinity of the beam rises. Air
mass subsequently flows away from the beam center (at the
speed of sound) lowering the index of refraction. The
beam then experiences a weak defocusing effect much the
same as a negative lens. Frequently an annular irradiance
distribution appears in some planes away from the transmitter plane. This has been demonstrated experimentally
and typical results are shown in Fig. 16 (frame two, num-
bered from left to right, and top to bottom). These

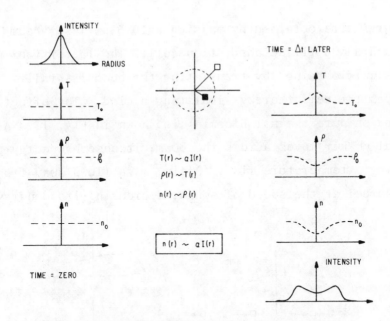

Fig. 15.   Simplified graphical description of thermal blooming in quiescent air.

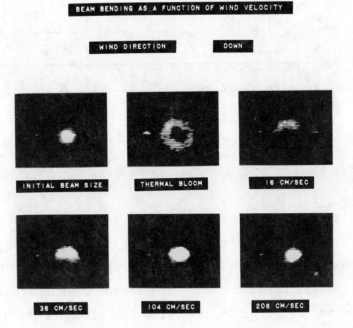

Fig. 16.   Experimental data describing thermal blooming and beam bending for various transverse wind speeds.

pictures were obtained by passing a 10.6 μm laser beam
through a CO_2 filled absorption cell. The latter four pictures were obtained by translating the beam laterally
through the cell thereby simulating a wind. The effect of
a wind on pure thermal blooming is shown in Fig. 17. As a
parcel of air moves across the beam, it absorbs energy
causing a temperature rise. Again, mass flows away from
the parcel at the speed of sound, decreasing its density.

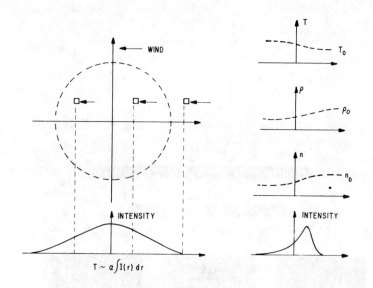

Fig. 17. *Simplified graphical description of thermal beam
bending for a constant transverse wind.*

As a result, the density and therefore refractive index
profile across the beam both tend to decrease from the up-
wind to the downwind side. The light rays, bending into
more (optically) dense regions, are therefore refracted
into the wind. In Fig. 16, the wind direction is downward
in frames 3 to 6. Note that for slower wind speeds a
crescent shaped irradiance distribution occurs. At higher

wind speeds, the parcel of air is carried through the beam
so rapidly that very little energy can be deposited during
the time that it is in the vicinity of the beam. Density
changes are thus very small, and consequently, very little
optical distortion occurs. The transit time of a parcel
of air across the beam is a characteristic time of interest
to the thermal blooming problem. For times less than this
number, thermal blooming (beam divergence in frame 2 of
Fig. 16) is the main source of optical distortion. For
times long compared to the transit time, a steady state
irradiance distribution evolves.

Another characteristic time of importance to thermal blooming is the sound speed transit time across the
beam (also called the acoustic transit time, t_{ac}). Temperature disturbances in a gas cause pressure disturbances
that are rapidly dispersed as sound waves. At STP, the
speed of sound is approximately 330 m/sec. In times long
compared to the acoustic transit time, the isobaric assumption of the hydrodynamic processes is valid. In times
short compared to this, computation of transient density
changes is no longer isobaric and requires special treatment. This is a time regime of interest in high energy
laser pulse propagation.

For the record, the parabolic wave equations is
generally used for the thermal blooming problem

$$\nabla_T^2 U - 2ikn_o \frac{\partial U}{\partial Z} + k^2(n^2 - n_o^2)U = 0, \qquad (33)$$

where $[U \exp(-ikn_o Z)]$ is the solution of the reduced wave
equation. Second derivatives of U in the propagation

direction (Z) have been dropped in Eq. (33). The index of refraction difference term $(n^2 - n_o^2)$ is approximated well by $2n_o n_1$, where $n = n_o + n_1$, n_o being the index of refraction of the quiescent gas (for air $n_o \simeq 1.000292$). Using either the Gladstone-Dale relation for gases or the Lorentz-Lorenz relationship, one gets $n_1 = (n_o - 1) \rho_1/\rho_o$, where density has been written as $\rho = \rho_o + \rho_1$, ρ_o being the quiescent gas density.

The density perturbation for the case of a constant transverse wind, v_o, can be determined by linearizing the appropriate hydrodynamic equations. Under the assumption that $v_o \ll c_\infty$ where c_∞ is the speed of sound in the gas, the process can be shown to be isobaric. The density perturbations are given by

$$\frac{\rho_1(x,y,z)}{\rho_o} = - \frac{(\gamma-1)}{\gamma\, v_o\, p_o} \int_{x-v_o t}^{x} dx' \; \rho_o \dot{Q}(x',y,z) \;, \quad (34)$$

where $\rho_o \dot{Q}(x,y,z)$ is the laser heat deposition term. p_o is the ambient pressure, and is taken as constant in this analysis. Time (t) is measured from the instant the laser is turned on, though the solution is really only valid for times long compared to the acoustic transit time. In steady state $(t \to \infty)$, the lower limit of the integral can be set to minus infinity.

The heat deposition term is a function of the radiation wavelength and its specific atomic or molecular absorption-thermalization process in air. If pure, instantaneous heating is assumed (as is the case for absorption of 10.6 μm radiation by water), Eq. (34) is just

$$\frac{\rho_1(\vec{r})}{\rho_o} = -\left(\frac{\gamma-1}{\gamma}\right)\frac{\alpha}{v_o\,p_o}\int_{-\infty}^{x}I(x',y,z)\,dx' \tag{35}$$

where α is the absorption coefficient for the specific absorption-thermalization process being considered.

For the case of 10.6 µm radiation, carbon dioxide in addition to water vapor is also found to be a strong absorber in the atmosphere. The absorption process is between the lower and upper lasing vibrational energy levels ($10°0$ and $00°1$). The vibrational energy level diagram which is important to the absorption of 10.6 µm radiation by CO_2 is shown in Fig. 18. Briefly, the absorption energetics are the following.[43] Upon absorption of a photon of 10.6 µm radiation, the CO_2 vibrational system is raised from the ($10°0$) state to the ($00°1$) energy level. To raise a CO_2 molecule to this level, energy ε_{001} must be added to the system. A portion of this energy comes from the 10.6 µm photon, the remaining portion coming from the energy in the ($10°0$) vibrational level (ε_{100}). The ($10°0$) energy level is now no longer in thermal equilibrium and therefore, through collisional deactivation, it is repopulated by taking energy out of the translational energy (temperature) reservoir. The process is very quick and engenders an immediate decrease in the temperature of the gas. Of course, this condition cannot last forever. Energy has been absorbed by the gas, and ultimately there must occur a temperature rise. This occurs in the following way. The ($00°1$) level of CO_2 is in near equilibrium with the first vibrational energy level of nitrogen. In the atmosphere there is roughly 2600 times as many nitrogen systems as CO_2 systems. Through collisional

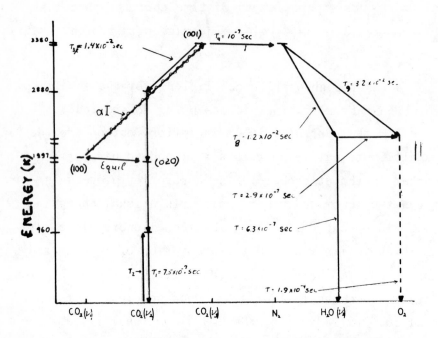

Fig. 18. *Vibrational energy level diagram of molecular*
species important to the kinetic processes of
CO_2 *absorption of 10.6 μm radiation (Ref. 43).*

deactivation, most of the energy stored in the (00°1) CO_2
systems is quickly transferred to the nitrogen systems.
The reverse reaction is effectively much slower because of
the preponderance of the nitrogen molecules to carbon dioxide molecules. The excited nitrogen atoms can also return
to ground through collisional deactivation with H_2O or O_2.
All these rates are slow, however, producing in effect a
freezing of the energy in the nitrogen vibrational energy
reservoir. Thus until nitrogen releases its energy, the
effect of absorption of 10.6 μm radiation by CO_2 is to cool
the air. In the case of a wind, the extent to which a parcel of air is cooled or heated by the CO_2 absorption

process depends on the length of time that the parcel is
in the beam and the net relaxation rate of nitrogen.

Considering the two main sources of 10.6 μm
absorption (H_2O and CO_2), one can obtain for the density
variation of Eq. (35)

$$\frac{\rho_1(\vec{r})}{\rho_o} = -\alpha\left(\frac{\gamma-1}{\gamma}\right) \cdot \frac{1}{v_o \rho_o} \int_{-\infty}^{x} \left\{ 1 - \sigma\exp\left[-\frac{(x-x')}{v_o \tau}\right]\right\}$$

$$\times \quad I(x',y,z)\,dx' \,, \qquad\qquad (36)$$

where

$$I(x,y,z) = \text{irradiance distribution of the laser}$$

$$\tau = \text{net relaxation rate of nitrogen}$$

$$\alpha = \alpha_{H_2O} + \alpha_{CO_2}$$

$$\sigma = \left(\frac{\varepsilon_{001}}{\varepsilon_{001} - \varepsilon_{100}}\right)\frac{\alpha_{CO_2}}{\alpha} \simeq 2.441\,\frac{\alpha_{CO_2}}{\alpha} \,.$$

Note that when $\tau = 0$, then $\frac{\rho_1}{\rho_o} < 0$; i.e., no cooling can
occur. Similarly, if $\alpha_{CO_2} \simeq 0$, then $\sigma \simeq 0$ and again no cooling can occur. In general neither of these conditions
occurs in practice, so that the integrand of Eq. (36) may,
under the appropriate conditions, assume negative values,
thus indicating a cooling phenomenon. Sigma (σ) assumes
its largest value (2.441) when $\alpha_{H_2O} \simeq 0$, so that the
kinetic cooling phenomenon (as it is sometimes called) can

be expected to occur at the higher altitudes in the
atmosphere where the water vapor content is small.
Finally, it is clear that no kinetic cooling can occur if
$\alpha_{H_2O} > 1.44\ \alpha_{CO_2}$, though partial cooling can offset to some
degree the heating due to absorption by H_2O.

Prior to the full diffraction treatment of thermal
blooming [Eq. (28)], extensive work on this subject was
also performed using geometrical optics.[39,44,45] The full
diffraction approach to the problem was later found necessary however, in order to adequately describe focused
beams and cases of severe ray deflections (leading to caus-
tics in geometrical optics).

Figure 19 is an example calculation of a diffraction
code. The results are typical of focused beams with a
constant transverse wind. Pure heating is assumed. Notice
that the beam is deflected into the wind, and that a crescent, or sugar scoop irradiance profile develops. The amplitude in each frame has been normalized to unity. Again,
I reiterate these are steady state results (i.e., the beam
is assumed to have been in for a long period of time).

The inclusion of kinetic cooling in the calculations
can dramatically alter the focal plane irradiance distribution. For example, in Fig. 20, a typical focal plane
irradiance distribution is seen when $\tau = 0$ (pure heating).
In Fig. 21, the same case is shown when $\tau = 15$ msec. With
kinetic cooling present, the beam is seen to deflect downwind, develop an irradiance distribution which appears to
be self-trapping to some degree, and exhibit a peak irradiance which is better than twice as large as for the purely
heating case. This latter characteristic, in fact, seems
to be generally true. Whenever any degree of kinetic

cooling is present, far field maximum irradiance values are always improved over the comparable pure thermal blooming case.

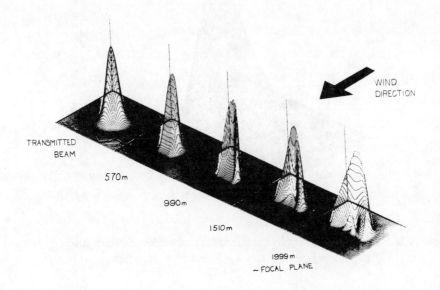

Fig. 19. *Typical example of a theoretical computer calculation of thermal blooming (Ref. 36).*

In this vein, however, I should point out that Sica[46] at NRL has recently found experimentally that the earlier published values for the nitrogen relaxation rate are too large. Specifically, in the limit of very little water content, Sica's experimental measurements tend to agree with the theoretical published values. However, for larger water vapor levels, the published values appear to be much as 6 times larger than the experimental measurements. Generally speaking, however, for high altitude propagation, this does not noticeably alter any previous conclusions because there is usually a sharp decrease in water vapor content with altitude (see Fig. 22).

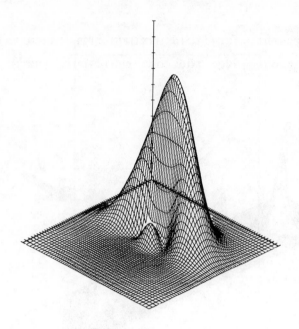

Fig. 20.   *Characteristic thermal blooming irradiance profile for a purely heating medium.*

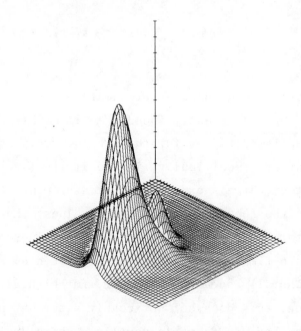

Fig. 21.   *Characteristic kinetic cooling irradiance profile for a dominately cooling medium. Wind is in same direction for both Fig. 20 and 21.*

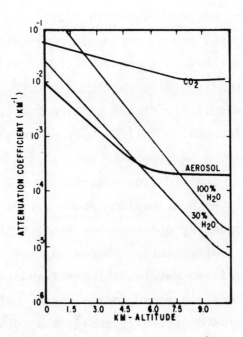

Fig. 22. Attenuation of 10.6 µm radiation in the air (Ref. 43).

Results And Studies Developed From The Basic Problem

In dealing with nonlinear problems, one of the most difficult tasks is arriving at good scaling laws. By doing this, however, one can circumvent the usual time-consuming operation of numerical integration of Eq. (34) for each and every specific case of interest.

To approach such a problem one must know the parametric dependencies of the specific variables of interest. Analysis of the governing equations frequently helps, but since the process is nonlinear, some care must be exercised with this approach. In this section, I describe some studies which have been conducted to investigate the parametric dependencies of thermal blooming.

Power Optimization--Solving Eq. (33), one finds that
with increasing output power, the maximum irradiance in the
receiver plane first begins to increase, gradually saturates and then actually begins to decrease with yet larger
power. This characteristic of the problem has lead to a
group of parametric studies called power optimization
curves. In Fig. 23, a sample power optimation study is
shown with results obtained from numerically solving Eq.
(33). Notice that the peak maximum power varies sharply,
as does the corresponding optimum power setting for different absorption coefficients. Note also that these
curves are for one fixed wavelength, one fixed transmitting
aperture diameter and one fixed focal length. Altering
any of these can also drastically change the location
(total output power) and magnitude of the focal plane maximum power.

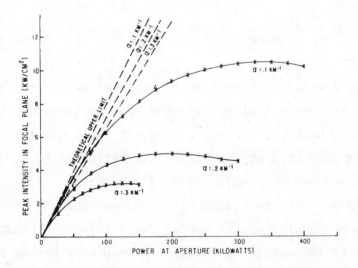

*Fig. 23.   Thermal blooming power optimization curves
          (John Hayes, NRL, 1973).*

Studying curves like these, Hayes and other at NRL were able to reliably fit all computed calculations for a fixed wavelength and aperture size to a function of the form

$$I_{peak} (f) = \tag{37}$$

$$\frac{I_{vac} (f) \, e^{-\alpha f}}{1 + A(\alpha, f) \left(\dfrac{\alpha P_T}{v_o} e^{-\alpha f} \right) + B(\alpha, f) \left(\dfrac{\alpha P_T}{v_o} e^{-\alpha f} \right)^2},$$

where $A(\alpha, f)$ and $B(\alpha, f)$ are polynomial functions in α and f (f is the focal length). The solid line in Fig. 23 is the parametric curve obtained with Eq. (37). From a consideration of the form of Eq. (36), one can deduce that blooming should scale in some fashion with quantities like $(\alpha P_T / v_o)$ and (αz). This is clearly reflected in Eq. (37).

Other parameters which appear in the analysis and may be good scaling quantities are

$$\frac{f}{2\omega} = f/\text{number}$$

$$\frac{\pi \omega^2}{\lambda f} = \text{Fresnel Number}$$

$$N_F = (n_o - 1) \left(\frac{\gamma - 1}{\gamma} \right) \left(\frac{\alpha \, P_T}{v_o} \right) \left(\frac{z^2}{p_o \omega_1{}^3} \right) \left(\frac{\omega_1}{\omega_f} \right) \qquad *$$

* a dimensionless parameter developed first by Gebhardt and Smith (Ref. 38).

   Parametric Dependence on Transmitted Beam Diameter
and Wavelength--To deduce other scaling laws, one needs to
study the additional effects of apertures and radiation
wavelength on the thermal blooming process. Figure 24 is
an example of the wavelength dependence of the process.
Holding all else constant for each curve (α, ω, P_T, f, v_o),
the wavelength of the radiation source was varied. The
dashed curve shows the ideal limit of maximum irradiance
versus wavelength. The solid curves lying below this are
for different absorption coefficients. For ($\alpha P_T/v_o$) $\geq$
0.9 watts-sec/m^2, the curves show an increase in focal
plane irradiance with decreasing wavelength at a rate that
is much less than the theoretical limit of λ^{-2}. In Fig.
25 the same data (normalized to the vacuum intensity) plus
other data as well, are plotted (on log-log scales). The
limiting slope for decreasing wavelength is seen to be
$\sim$ 1.54. Since $I_o(\lambda) \sim \lambda^{-2}$, then for this set of conditions, one can conclude that $I_{max} \sim \lambda^{-.46}$, when $\alpha \geq$
5×10^{-5} m^{-1}. Note that Fig. 25 shows data for other
transmitter aperture sizes as well, and that all the data
reflects the above wavelength dependence.

   In a similar fashion, Fig. 26 shows a parametric
study of transmitting aperture dependence. Again the
dashed line is the theoretical limit increasing as ω^2.
The thermal blooming results lie below this curve, and
show an interesting result. As the transmitter aperture
is increased, the focal plane irradiance in the presence
of thermal blooming increases with an aperture dependence
much the same as the aperture dependence of the vacuum
propagation case. Figure 27 is a log-log plot of the
relative irradiance, and shows a slope of approximately

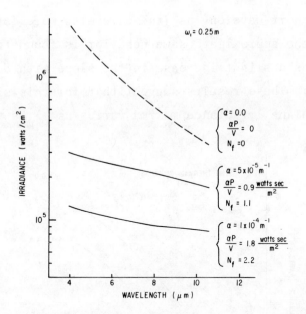

Fig. 24. Wavelength dependence of thermal blooming.
Absolute irradiance (peak) in focal plane.

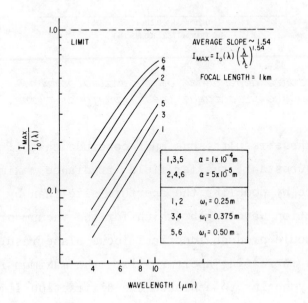

Fig. 25. Wavelength dependence of thermal blooming.
Relative irradiance (peak) in focal plane.

0.5. For short wavelengths (these results were for λ =
10.6 µm), the approximate same behavior is found to occur,
with perhaps a slight increase in the slope with decreasing
wavelength. These results suggest that for this situation,
the focal plane irradiance maxima varies as $I_{max} \sim \omega^{2 \cdot 5}$.

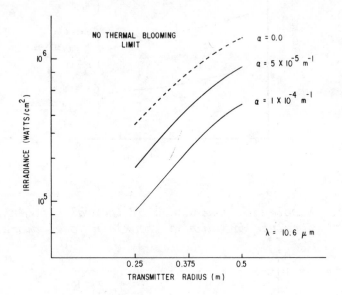

NO THERMAL BLOOMING LIMIT

$a = 0.0$

$a = 5 \times 10^{-5}$ m^{-1}

$a = 1 \times 10^{-4}$ m^{-1}

IRRADIANCE (WATTS/cm^2)

$\lambda = 10.6$ µm

TRANSMITTER RADIUS (m)

*Fig. 26. Aperture dependence of thermal blooming.
Absolute irradiance (peak) in focal plane.*

From these results, one must conclude that if all
else is held constant, the far field irradiance maximum is
increased more by doubling the aperture size than by halv-
ing the radiation wavelength (which for the vacuum propagation case would produce identical focal plane results).
In fact, with increasing aperture size, the maximum irradiance actually begins to approach the diffraction limited
irradiance whereas with decreasing wavelength, the maximum
irradiance actually diverges from the limiting value. The
reason for this behavior is two-fold. Firstly, the shorter

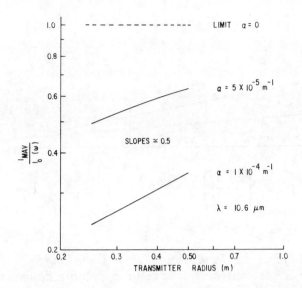

Fig. 27. *Aperture dependence of thermal blooming.*
Relative irradiance (peak) in focal plane.

wavelength radiation is affected more strongly by comparable density gradients (as with turbulence) than the
longer wavelength radiation. Secondly, the shorter wavelength radiation exhibits spot sizes at all points along
the beam that are, in the vacuum limit, smaller than the
longer wavelength spot sizes (for the same transmitter
diameter, of course). Therefore, for a constant output
power, higher intensity levels result. This is true also
for larger aperture systems for planes near the focal
plane. However, at the other planes along the propagation
axis that are slightly removed from the focal plane, the
shorter wavelength system, at fixed transmitting aperture
size, still has larger irradiance values than a longer
wavelength system operating with very large transmitting
optics. The situation is shown in Fig. 28, where the
shorter wavelength (λ_1) and larger aperture size (ω_2) have

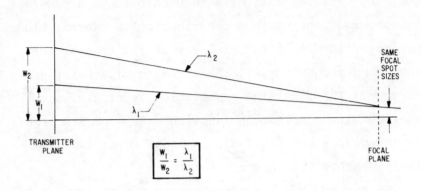

*Fig. 28. Simplified explanation of the wavelength
dependence and transmitting aperture dependence
on thermal blooming.*

been chosen to make the focal plane vacuum spot sizes the
same for the two beams (i.e., $\lambda_1/\lambda_2 = \omega_1/\omega_2$). Thermal
blooming is a nonlinear process that is driven solely by
the form and magnitude of the laser beam irradiance distribution. Hence, one would therefore expect that for two
vacuum equivalent systems (focal plane irradiance distributions), one with a large aperture and the other with a
short radiation wavelength, that less thermal blooming
would occur in the former case.

A related subject pertaining to this problem is the
following. What portion of the propagation path contributes most to the thermal blooming phenomenon? In general,
this is a complex question, the answer depending strongly
on all the parameters. However, some things can be con-
cluded. First, for a collimated beam (or diverging beam)
it is easy to show that the maximum weight occurs at the
transmitter. Here the density gradients are the largest
and the propagation level arm (to any observation plane)

the longest. For the case of a focused beam in a *constant*
transverse wind, the maximum contribution to thermal blooming no longer occurs in the vicinity of the transmitter.
Two competing mechanisms, 1) the strength of density gradients and 2) the remaining propagation level arm, move
the maximum of the weighting function away from the transmitter and nearer the focal plane--and I might add sur-
prisingly near to the latter.

One can do a number of things to try to study this
problem, but I think one of the clearest presentations of
the effect can be seen if the following is computed. Consider a slice of propagation path which is, say, 1/5 or
1/10 the total path length. Make this slice of path
absorbing with some absorption coefficient α. Specify
the rest of the propagation path to have a zero absorption
coefficient (i.e., free space). Now place the absorbing
segment at different positions between the transmitter and
receiver and note the reduction in maximum irradiance. In
Fig. 29, I show the results of performing this computation
with a segment 200 meters long; the focal length was 1 km
and transmitting aperture diameter was 30 cm. The abscis-
sa locates the center of the segment along the propagation path and the ordinate presents the obtained relative
irradiance for each case. The greatest reduction in
irradiance occurs for a segment located between 700 and
800 meters. Shortening the segment length to 100 meters
improves the resolution of this process, and these results
are shown in Fig. 30. Apparently, the maximum weighting
occurs near the 800 m point. To check our understanding
of this process, I considered a similar arrangement with
a smaller transmitting aperture diameter of 20 cm. The

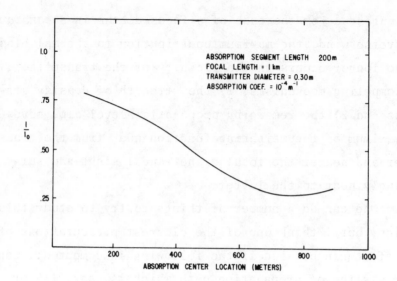

Fig. 29.   *Relative path contribution to the irradiance*
degradation caused by thermal blooming.

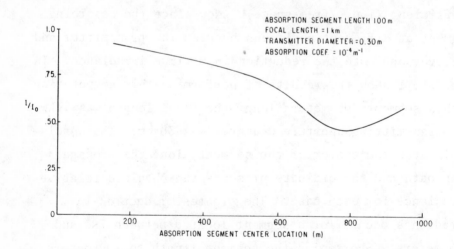

Fig. ⠀   *Relative path contribution to the irradiance*
degradation caused by thermal blooming.

maximum of the weighting function should move toward the
transmitter, and it does (see Fig. 31). I must point out,

however, that the difficulty with using this sort of an
analysis to locate the maximum weighting location is that
the effects of accumulated optical distortions are not
accurately assessed. Other work I have done seems to indicate that for each of these cases a better estimate of
the location of the weighting function maxima is actually
slightly closer to the transmitter. Nonetheless, the conclusion is that for a focused beam, the portion of the
optical path that contributes most heavily to the thermo-
optical distortions is well away from the transmitter
plane, and in particular, for larger aperture transmitting
systems, the position moves closer and closer to the
receiver plane. This result obviously has some bearing
on the explanation of the wavelength versus transmitter
aperture size dependencies.

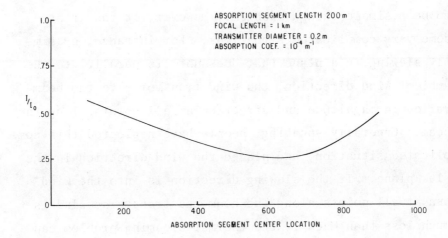

*Fig. 31. Relative path contribution to the irradiance
degradation caused by thermal blooming.*

With the inclusion of slewing, wavelength dependent
absorption coefficients, etc., the preceding discussions

must be somewhat re-evaluated. Nevertheless, the approach
taken and some of the typical dependencies of the various
parameters entering in the thermal blooming problem should
be clear. Generally speaking, the problem is very complex,
and is made even more so by the necessity to treat special
problems and effects which often occur.

Special Problems In Thermal Blooming

A number of interesting but specialized problems
have developed as a result of the basic thermal blooming
problem. One of the most obvious variations to the basic
problem is the inclusion of an angular slewing velocity
which has the effect of varying the transverse wind speed
at points along the beam. At first thought, this seems
to be a simple enough problem. However, it can create
some very complicated situations. For instance, by simply slewing in a plane that does not lie parallel to the
ambient wind direction, the wind transverse to the beam
varies in magnitude and direction at all points along the
beam. Generally speaking, people have neglected this complicated situation, and placed the wind direction in the
slew plane. If the slewing direction is into the wind
and at all points along the beam the transverse wind is
much less than Mach 1, the thermal blooming problem can
be treated quite well with a simple modification to the
basic problem, namely by varying the transverse wind speed
with range along the beam. However, two other problems of
infinitely more complexity can occur if 1) the slew direction is reversed, and 2) if the slew rate is very large
giving rise to transonic winds transverse to the beam.

In the first case, if conditions are right, the slewing
induced wind and the naturally occurring wind can cancel
one another, producing a situation where the wind transverse to the beam is zero.[47] These are called "stagnation
zones." Analysis of the wind flow in the vicinity of
stagnation zones is complex and accurate computer modeling
of even the simplest problems is very difficult (and
approximate). Assuming that the air in the stagnation
zone is truly stationary (which it usually is not) and
making some assumptions with regard to the way in which
the density gradients are modeled in this region, I
obtained the irradiance distribution for a beam that has
been on for 100 msec (the stagnation zone density variation growth is time dependent) shown in Fig. 32. The density gradient in the stagnation region acts like a negative lens, spreading the beam in all directions. In this
case, the focusing effect of thermal blooming along the
wind axis prevents the total divergence of the beam in
that direction, thus resulting in a focal plane irradiance
distribution that is doubly peaked in the direction normal
to the wind. The strength of the effect varies like
$(\alpha P/v_o \omega_1)$ for times longer than the acoustic transit time,
though it is mitigated somewhat by the motion of the stagnation zone in space, or if it is not moving, then by the
initiation of an induced convection wind, or both.

The second situation, that of a transonic flow, is a
relatively new problem and is still being investigated.[48,49,50]
The nature of the process can be visualized by looking at
Fig. 33. Assume that at $t = 0$, the beam is in the position
shown. The medium is continually absorbing energy, and
therefore (approximately) cylindrical sound waves are

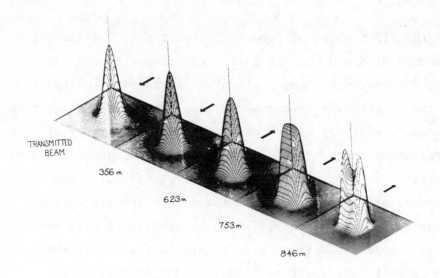

TRANSMITTED
BEAM

356 m

623m

753m

846m

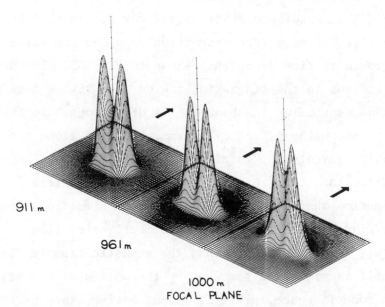

911 m

961m

1000 m
FOCAL PLANE

*Fig. 32.   Thermal optical effects of a high energy beam
            propagating through a stagnation zone.*

constantly being generated. At $t = \Delta t$, the sound waves
generated at $t = 0$ have reached the position shown by the
dashed lines. At that time, the beam has reached the
position shown. The intersection of the beam and the

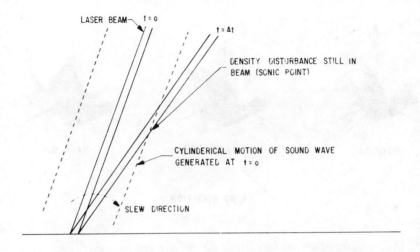

Fig. 33. *Simplified graphical description of the source*
          of optical degradation arising from trans-sonic
          winds.

sound wave locates the position of transverse sonic wind
flow. The result is that at this point in the beam, density perturbations grow into a shock wave across the leading edge of the beam. Depending on the nature of the
medium and radiation, cooling or heating might be the
dominant temperature effect. Whichever is the case, an
underpressure or overpressure shock wave, respectively,
develops. Figure 34 shows three (3) density profiles, one
at Mach 1.1, Mach 1.0, and Mach 0.9, respectively, from
left to right. The first and the last profiles are steady
state solutions obtained from a two-dimensional hydro-code
under the assumption of a gaussian shaped irradiance distribution (kinetic cooling dominated this case). The
middle picture was obtained for the same conditions at a
velocity of Mach 1. It is not a steady state solution,
and is found to grow (after some initial millisecond
transients) linearly in time. In Fig. 34 the plots are

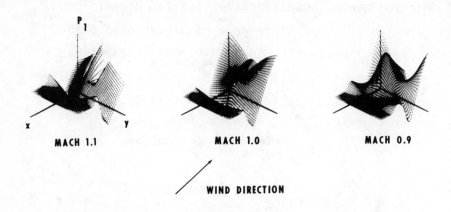

*Fig. 34.   Computer calculations of density profiles
            generated by a high energy beam with trans-
            sonic transverse winds.*

all normalized and consequently do not reflect the true
relative magnitudes of the density gradients. Generally
speaking, for a given time the density variations are
always larger for the Mach 1 case than for velocities
greater than or less than this. One finds that for velocity ranges other than Mach 1, the steady state density
profile evolves in a time long compared to $2\ \omega(z)/\left|v_o-c_\infty\right|$,
where the bars denote absolute value, and where $\omega(z)$ is
the beam radius at the position z where v_o is the
transverse wind. Using these density profiles, I modeled
a propagation configuration in which the Mach 1 velocity
point occurred in the center of a 1 km path. The time
evolution of the focal plane irradiance distribution is
shown in Fig. 35 for a time up to 100 msec. In each frame
the maximum irradiance has been scaled to unity.

    Another class of problems deals with the effects of
nongaussian and/or nonideal phase profiles on thermal
blooming. This category includes the study of apertured

and obscured beams, nondiffraction limited beams,[51] and
beams propagating in the presence of atmospheric turbulence. Work is presently under way in all these areas.
The problems are difficult, with the order of difficulty,
I believe, increasing as listed, respectively. Time does
not permit a discussion of these problem areas.

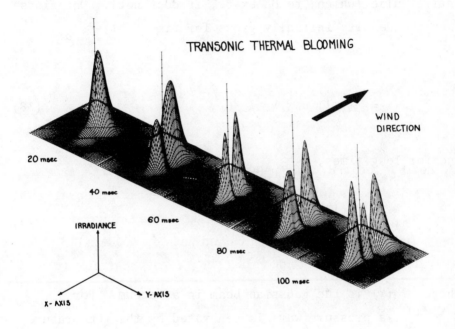

TRANSONIC THERMAL BLOOMING

WIND
DIRECTION

IRRADIANCE

20 msec

40 msec

60 msec

80 msec

100 msec

Y-AXIS

X-AXIS

Fig. 35. A simulation of optical effects for a beam
propagating through a trans-sonic region.

Finally, there is the problem of short pulse propagation. Here one is concerned with pulse lengths whose
duration is on the order of the hydrodynamic times, i.e.,
on the order of the acoustic transit time. The problem
describes thermal blooming in the transient time regime.
This was purposely avoided in the treatment of the original
basic thermal blooming problem. To simplify things

slightly, it is usually assumed that during the pulse, the transverse motion of the air is negligible; that is, we assume the wind is zero, and thereby treat a cylindrically symmetric problem. The hydrodynamics can be solved exactly (for the linearized equations) if the irradiance distribution is assumed to remain gaussian in shape throughout the entire pulse (which, to be exact, it does not). One finds that the density initially grows for time[52] $t \ll t_{ac}$ ($t_{ac} = \omega/c_\infty$) as

$$\rho_1 = (\gamma-1) \alpha t^3 \nabla^2 I_o/6 , \tag{38}$$

and for long times, $t \gg t_{ac}$, like

$$\rho_1 = \frac{-(\gamma-1) \alpha t I_o}{c_\infty^2} \tag{39}$$

where $I_o(r)$ is the gaussian beam in a vacuum. For $t \ll t_{ac}$, a pressure wave is generated by the temperature rise (drop) which then propagates as an acoustic disturbance away from (towards) the beam. For times $t \gg t_{ac}$, the pressure is found to be constant, and the usual isobaric density growth occurs. In Fig. 36, one can see the propagation of the overpressure out of the beam (pure heating case), the later density changes being linear in t and proportional to the assumed irradiance profile of the laser (gaussian).

For sufficiently high energy pulses, serious optical distortions can result. Figure 37 reproduces some of the results of Ulrich and Wallace[52] for the propagation of

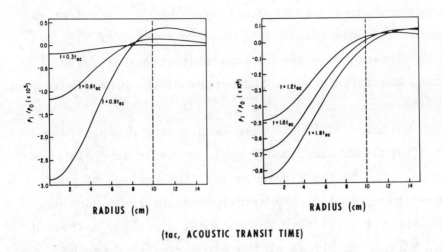

Fig. 36. Transient density growth caused by a pulse of high energy laser radiation (Ref. 36).

a pulsed collimated beam. The range z is in units of Rayleigh range $(\pi\omega^2_{tr}/\lambda)$, and times in fractions of t_{ac}. The results can be explained as follows. As air mass is moved out of the center of the beam in the compression wave, the local index of refraction decreases. Rays in the center of the beam are bent outward, redistributing the

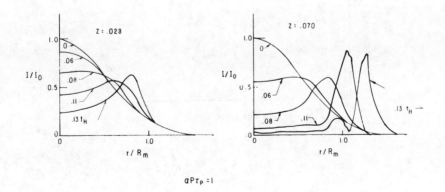

Fig. 37. Blooming of a pulsed, collimated beam (Ref. 52).

energy very quickly in an annulous shape. This effect was
seen for the case where $t \gg t_{ac}$ in frame 2 of Fig. 16.
For the longer range the optical distortions are more
severe, the irradiance in the center of the beam almost
going to zero.

Ulrich[53,54,55] has also studied the propagation of
pulsed, focused beams, and a typical result is shown in
Fig. 38. The bottom figure is the time average of the
upper figure results. Apparently a donut irradiance distribution can still form in the focal plane for a focused
beam, but the magnitude of the outer ring seems to be
reduced over the collimated beam result.

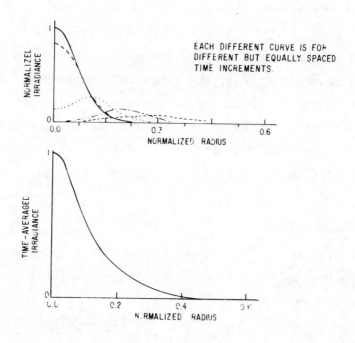

Fig. 38. Blooming of a pulsed, focused beam (Ref. 54).

Ulrich has noted (personal communication) that for
the case of pulsed, focused laser beams, the region along

the propagation path which contributes most substantially
to the thermo-optical distortions is near the focal plane.
There are two reasons for this. One is that in this region, the density perturbations are the strongest, owing
to the higher irradiance values obtained by focusing. The
second reason is that because the beam is smaller (in diameter) here, the acoustic waves can be more rapidly propagated away from the beam, resulting in a more rapid density
perturbation growth. Thus even though the propagation
lever arm is very short for these index of refraction disturbances, their magnitude is so strong that serious optical effects are still observed. Interestingly enough,
this is in agreement with the earlier discussion of the
range dependence of steady state thermal blooming.

REFERENCES

1. V. I. Tatarski, *Wave Propagation in a Turbulent Medium*,
   Dover Publications, Inc., New York (1961).

2. L. A. Chernov, *Wave Propagation in a Random Medium*,
   McGraw-Hill Book Company, Inc., New York (1960).

3. V. I. Tatarski, *The Effects of the Turbulent Atmosphere
   on Wave Propagation*, Israel Program for Scientific
   Translations, Jerusalem, available from US Dept. of
   Commerce (1971).

4. J. W. Strohbehn, *Proc. IEEE*, 56, 1301 (1968).

5. R. S. Lawrence and J. W. Strohbehn, *Proc. IEEE*, 58,
   1523 (1970).

6. R. S. Lawrence, G. R. Ochs and S. F. Clifford, *JOSA*,
   60, 826 (1970).

7. G. R. Ochs, *Measurements of 0.63 μm Laser-Beam Scin-tillation in Strong Atmospheric Turbulence*, ESSA Tech. Report ERL 154-WPL 10 (1969).

8. G. R. Ochs and R. S. Lawrence, *JOSA*, 59, 226 (1969).

9. J. R. Kerr, *JOSA*, 62, 1040 (1972).

10. G. R. Ochs and R. S. Lawrence, *JOSA*, 59, 226 (1969).

11. G. R. Ochs, R. R. Bergman and J. R. Snyder, *Lett. JOSA*, 59, 231 (1969).

12. A. Ishimaru, *Proc. IEEE*, 57, 407 (1969).

13. R. F. Lutomirski and H. T. Yura, *Appl. Opt.* 10, 1652 (1971).

14. H. T. Yura, *JOSA*, 63, 107 (1973).

15. H. T. Yura, *JOSA*, 63, 567 (1973).

16. G. R. Heidbreder, *IEEE*, *PGAP*, 15, 90 (1967).

17. J. P. Moreland and S. A. Collins, *JOSA*, 59, 10 (1969).

18. D. L. Fried, *JOSA*, 56, 3172 (1966).

19. R. E. Hufnagel and N. R. Stanley, *JOSA*, 54, 52 (1964).

20. S. A. Collins, Jr. and E. K. Damon, *Angle of Arrival Calculations at 10.6 μm*, RADC-TR-71-124 (1971).

21. J. R. Kerr and R. Eiss, *JOSA*, 62, 682 (1972).

22. J. Dowling and P. M. Livingston, *Behavior of Focused Beams in Atmospheric Turbulence: Measurements and Comments on the Theory*, to be published, July 1973.

23. J. R. Kerr and J. R. Dunphy, *JOSA*, 63, 1 (1973).

24. R. J. Hull, T. J. Gilmartin and L. C. Marquet, *Laser Beam Wander in Atmospheric Propagation*, Project Report LTP-7 (1971).

25. E. C. Alcarey and P. M. Livingston, *Measurements of the Beam Wander Phenomenon in a Turbulent Medium*, BRL-MR-2103 (1971).

26. T. Chiba, *Appl. Opt.*, 10, 2456 (1971).

27. D. L. Fried, *J. Opt. Soc. Am.*, <u>56</u> (1969).

28. D. L. Fried, *Proc. IEEE*, <u>55</u>, 57 (1967).

29. D. L. Fried and H. T. Yura, *Lett. to JOSA*, <u>62</u>, 600 (1972).

30. H. T. Yura, *Appl. Opt.*, <u>10</u>, 2771 (1971).

31. R. F. Lutomirski and H. T. Yura, *JOSA*, <u>61</u>, 482 (1971).

32. J. Wallace, *JOSA*, <u>62</u>, 373 (1972).

33. J. Wallace and M. Camac, *JOSA*, <u>60</u>, 1587 (1970).

34. J. N. Hayes, P. B. Ulrich and A. H. Aitken, *Appl. Opt.* <u>11</u>, 257 (1972).

35. P. M. Livingston, *Appl. Opt.* <u>10</u>, 426 (1971).

36. C. B. Hogge, *Thermo-Optical Effects of High Energy Laser Beams*, AFWL-TR-72-184 (1972).

37. D. C. Smith, *IEEE J. QE.* <u>5</u>, 6000 (1969).

38. F. G. Gebhardt and D. C. Smith, *Appl. Opt.* <u>11</u>, 244 (1972).

39. F. G. Gebhardt and D. C. Smith, *IEEE J. QE.* <u>7</u>, 63 (1971).

40. R. G. Buser and R. S. Rhode, *Appl. Opt.* <u>12</u>, 205 (1973).

41. J. R. Kenemuth, C. B. Hogge and P. V. Avizonis, *Appl. Phys. Lett.*, <u>17</u>, 220 (1970).

42. P. B. Ulrich, J. N. Hayes and A. H. Aitken, *JOSA*, <u>62</u>, 289 (1972).

43. A. D. Wood, M. Camac and E. T. Gerry, *Appl. Opt.* <u>10</u>, 1877 (1971).

44. P. V. Avizonis, C. B. Hogge, R. R. Butts, and J. R. Kenemuth, *Appl. Opt.* <u>11</u>, 554 (1972).

45. J. N. Hayes, *Appl. Opt.* <u>11</u>, 455 (1972).

46. L. Sica, *Interferometric Observations of Kinetic Cooling*, USNRL, to be published.

47. C. B. Hogge and R. R. Butts, *Propagation Effects of a Slewed Beam with Transverse Wind Null Spots*, AFWL-TR-73-76 (1973).

48. C. B. Hogge and J. E. Brau, *Optical Effects of Transonic and Supersonic Winds on High Energy Laser Beams*, AFWL-TR-73-131, Laser Division Spring Digest (1973).

49. J. E. Brau and C. B. Hogge, *A Comparison of One- and Two-Dimensional Models of Laser-Induced Density Anomalies in Flowing Air*, AFWL-TR-73-131, Laser Division Spring Digest (1973).

50. J. H. Hayes, *Thermal Blooming of Rapidly Slewed Laser Beams*, NRL Tech. Note (1973).

51. C. B. Hogge and M. Burlokoff, *Thermal Blooming of Nondiffraction Limited Beams*, AFWL-TR-73-77 (1973).

52. P. B. Ulrich and J. Wallace, *JOSA*, 63, 9 (1973).

53. P. B. Ulrich, *A Numerical Calculation of Thermal Blooming of Pulsed, Focused Laser Beams*, NRL Report 7382 (1971).

54. P. B. Ulrich, *Requirements for Experimental Verification of Thermal-Blooming Computer Results*, to appear *JOSA* (July 1973).

55. A. H. Aitken, J. H. Hayes and P. B. Ulrich, *Appl. Opt.* 12, 193 (1973).

CO_2 ELECTRICAL, CO_2 GAS DYNAMIC, HF CHEMICAL GAS LASERS
Petras Avizonis

5.1. INTRODUCTION

In considering high energy devices, the first thing
that comes to mind is the disposition of waste heat from
the lasing media. This waste energy occurs both from pumping and lasing action. Gas and liquid lasers have the
unique property of being able to exchange the active
medium,[1] thus getting rid of heat which is always delete-
rious to any high energy device. This process is described
by

$$\rho v_x C_p \frac{\partial T}{\partial x} + \frac{1}{r} \frac{\partial}{\partial r} rK \frac{\partial T}{\partial r} = Q \ .$$

Here T is the temperature, ρ is the density, C_p is the
heat capacity, K, the thermal conductivity, and Q is the
heat source. The first term is the rise in temperature
along the flow direction having velocity v_x. The second
term is the heat conduction by the gas to the walls. The
third term is the volumetric heat source. We can readily

see that if $v_x = 0$, all the heat has to be dissipated by
conduction. Since the heat source varies at least linearly with pressure (density), high pressure (high energy)
devices are immediately in trouble because of heat dissipation. On the other hand if the convective term dominates,
then at least the strongest (linear) pressure dependence of
Q cancels out. In order to control the temperature by
flow rather than by conduction, all that is required is
that the particle flow rate through the laser be fast compared with diffusion time of that particle from the center
of medium to the walls. This gives

$$\left(\frac{\rho C_p}{K}\right)\left(\frac{H}{2}\right)^2 >> \frac{L}{v_x} ,$$

where H is the height of the medium at right angles to
the flow, and L is the length of the lasing medium along
the flow. For all high energy gas lasers, this condition
has to be satisfied. In this chapter we discuss three such
lasers, namely, the electrical CO_2, the gas dynamic CO_2,
and the chemical HF lasers. We discuss them in the order
mentioned, not because this is the chronological order of
discovery, but because the latter two lasers have certain
technologies in common.

5.2.   ELECTRICAL CO_2 LASER

The CO_2-N_2 kinetic diagram is given in Fig. 1.[2-6]
We see that in an electron pumped laser system, both nitrogen and CO_2 are pumped at the rates k_4 and k_3 (for $00°1$

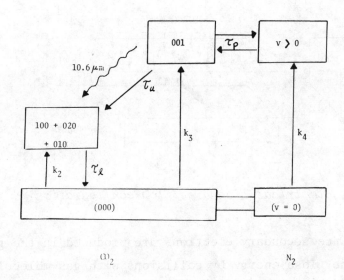

Fig. 1.　CO_2/N_2 kinetics schematic .

level of CO_2) respectively.　Also the lower levels of CO_2
can be electron collision pumped at the rate k_2.

　　A flowing electrical laser is implemented as shown
in Fig. 2.[7-9]　Gas flow is normal to the plane of the
paper.　Primary electrons are injected into the flow at
right angles to it and create secondary ionization through
the well known relationship

$$\frac{dn_e}{dt} = \sigma F N_o - \beta n_e^2 \ . \tag{1}$$

This equation simply states that secondary electron (n_e)
production depends on the pair production cross section　σ,
the primary electron beam flux　F, and the neutral gas
molecule density　N_o.　The electron loss occurs through
ion-electron recombination with a rate coefficient
$\beta \cong 10^{-7}$ cm^3/sec.

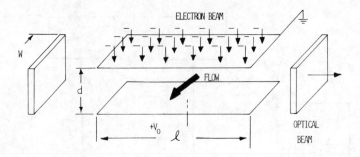

Fig. 2. Electrical discharge/flow configuration.

Once secondary electrons are produced in the gas
flow, they lose energy by collisions with gas molecules at
a rate proportional to the amount of pumping to the various
excited states. To make up for the loss, one needs to apply along the electron beam axis a DC electric field that
optimizes the secondary electron energy for pumping the N_2
and CO_2 upper levels. This field is the prime source of
pump energy. The pump rates[10,11] are plotted in Fig. 3 as
functions of electron energy. We see that the electron
energy t_e has to be maintained between 1.0 and 1.5 eV,
or else N_2 ionization becomes important. The various
pump rates for the CO_2-N_2 mixture are defined in
Fig. 1.

The next consideration is the removal of hot gas.
Figure 4 shows the upper (N_u/N_o) and lower (N_ℓ/N_o) population densities for three different gas temperatures. It
is evident that significant heating cannot be tolerated if
one wants to maximize the difference N_u-N_ℓ for a given
amount of pumping, defined in terms of the secondary electron density n_e. The equations governing these curves
will be developed shortly.

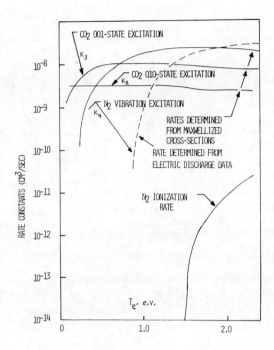

Fig. 3. Electron impact rate constants of interest in the N_2/CO_2 electric laser.

Referring back to Fig. 1 we see certain vibrational-vibrational (V-V) or vibrational-translation (V-T) energy exchange processes. First, there is the vibrational energy exchange rate[12-14] for transfer from N_2 to CO_2 (ψ_n/τ_p) and (ψ_c/τ_p) for transfer from CO_2 back to N_2. Here ψ_n and ψ_c are the mole fractions of N_2 and CO_2 respectively. The relaxation time (τ_p) for this process is shown in Fig. 5.

Next we have the vibrational-translational deactivation of the 00°1 (upper) CO_2 state by collisions with CO_2, N_2, and He.[12-14] Their respective rates are defined as ψ_c/τ_{uc}, ψ_h/τ_{uh}, ψ_n/τ_{un}, where ψ_h is the mole

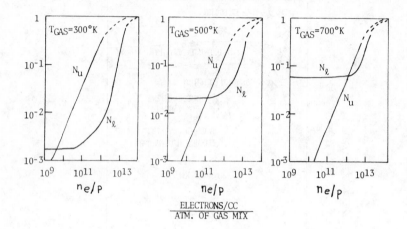

Fig. 4. *Excited-state populations in the $N_2/CO_2/He$ (2/1/3) discharge, indicating effects of gas temperatures and electron-impact excitation on gain.*

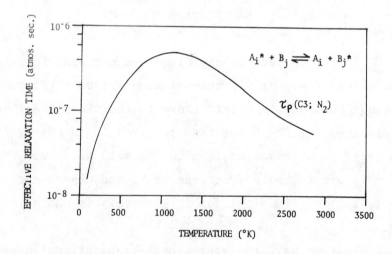

Fig. 5. *Effective relaxation times for single quantum inter-molecular vibration-vibration energy exchange between CO_2 (001) and N_2.*

fraction of He. This is depicted in Fig. 6 as a function
of temperature. Notice that we can write an "effective
$1/\tau_u$" rate as

$$1/\tau_u = \psi_n/\tau_{un} + \psi_h/\tau_{uh} + \psi_c/\tau_{uc} . \qquad (2)$$

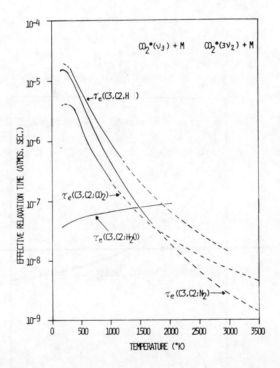

Fig. 6. *Effective relaxation times for 3 quanta intra-
molecular vibration-vibration energy exchange
between modes ν_3 and ν_2 of CO_2.*

Finally we need to consider the deactivation of the lower
laser level.[12-14] This is the primary role for He and its
temperature dependent rate is shown in Fig. 7. As before
we can write an "effective lower rate $1/\tau_\ell$" as a sum of

all deactivating collisions for the lower state, that is,

$$1/\tau_\ell = \psi_n/\tau_{\ell n} + \psi_h/\tau_{\ell h} + \psi_c/\tau_{\ell c} . \tag{3}$$

As is readily seen, He is the dominant species for the lower state deactivation. In addition it serves as a high capacity heat sink, (high C_p) minimizing the temperature rise in the gas.

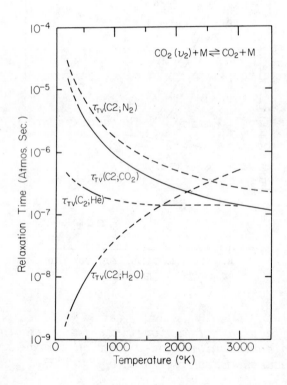

Fig. 7. Relaxation times for translation-vibration deactivation of mode ν_2 of CO_2.

We can now write the rate equations for the kinetic processes of an electrical CO_2 pulsed laser. We consider a time regime such that excitation and lasing pulses are shorter than the transit time of a gas molecule in the laser cavity. Therefore, the problem can be treated as a time dependent, rather than a position dependent, process. The equation of motion for excited nitrogen population N_n may be written as

$$\frac{dN_n}{dt} = k_4 N_n^0 n_e - \frac{\psi_c N_n}{\tau_p} + \frac{\psi_n N_u}{\tau_p} , \tag{4}$$

where the first term (on the right hand side) is the production of excited N_2 through electron pumping, the second term is the $V\text{-}V$ transfer to CO_2, and the third term is the $V\text{-}V$ transfer from CO_2 to N_2. The upper state CO_2 population has the equation of motion

$$\frac{dN_u}{dt} = k_3 N_c^0 n_e + \frac{\psi_c N_n}{\tau_p} - \frac{\psi_n N_u}{\tau_p} - \frac{N_u}{\tau_u} - \frac{\alpha I}{h\nu} . \tag{5}$$

Here, in the first right hand term, we have direct pumping of the upper state by electron collisions with ground state CO_2 (we assume that the ground state CO_2 is not depleted and is approximately equal to the total CO_2 concentration). The second and third terms represent $V\text{-}V$ energy transfer between N_2 and CO_2. The fourth term represents deactivation of the upper state by collisions, while the last term represents the radiative process with the saturated gain coefficient $\alpha = \sigma(N_u - N_\ell)$, the laser intensity I and the laser frequency ν. The lower state population has the time rate of change

$$\frac{dN_\ell}{dt} = \frac{\alpha I}{h\nu} + \frac{N_\ell}{\tau_\ell} + k_2 N_c^O n_e + \frac{N_c^O \exp[-h\nu/kT]}{\tau_\ell} \ . \tag{6}$$

This describes the filling by the radiative process, the upper state relaxation into the lower state, and the electron collision pumping, the depletion by V-T processes through collisions (primarily with Helium), and the equilibration with ground state through the reverse process.

Finally the time rate of change in temperature due to V-T processes is given by

$$\frac{dT}{dt} = \frac{h\nu_\ell}{C_\nu \rho_o} \left[\frac{N_\ell}{\tau_\ell} - \frac{N_c^O \exp(-h\nu/kT)}{\tau_\ell} \right] , \tag{7}$$

which is the difference between the heat release due to N_ℓ relaxation and the cooling of the media as the lower state is repopulated from the ground.

Before numerical solutions are actually developed, we can get an insight about some scaling parameters for such lasers. Consider the case where the pumping and deactivation has come to steady state with energy output. Then, we can set the time derivatives in Eqs. (4) through (6) to zero and combine (4) with (5). We obtain

$$(k_3 N_c^O + k_4 N_n^O) n_e - \frac{N_u}{\tau_u} = \frac{\alpha \bar{I}}{h\nu} \tag{8}$$

$$k_2 N_c^O n_e - \frac{N_\ell}{\tau_\ell} + \frac{N_c^O \exp[-h\nu/kT]}{\tau_\ell} = - \frac{\alpha \bar{I}}{h\nu}$$

in which $\bar{I}$ is the steady state intensity. For practical devices steady state may be reached after about 5 μsec of e-beam pumping.

Adding and subtracting Eq. (8), we find the relations

$$[(k_3 + k_2)N_c^O + k_4 N_n^O]n_e + \frac{N_c^O \exp[-h\nu/kT]}{\tau_\ell} = \frac{N_\ell}{\tau_\ell} + \frac{N_u}{\tau_u} \tag{9}$$

and

$$\frac{2\alpha\bar{I}}{h\nu} = [(k_3 - k_2)N_c^O + k_4 N_n^O]n_e \tag{10}$$

$$- \frac{N_u}{\tau_u} + \frac{N_\ell}{\tau_\ell} - \frac{N_c^O \exp[-h\nu/kT]}{\tau_\ell}.$$

Further recognizing that $\alpha = \sigma(N_u - N_\ell)$, we substitute $\alpha/\sigma - N_\ell$ for N_u and Eq. (9) for N_ℓ into (10). Assuming that the lower state electron pumping is small $(k_3 \gg k_2)$, we obtain the typical saturated gain coefficient for steady state:

$$\alpha = \frac{\sigma\left[\tau_u(k_3 N_c^O + k_4 N_n^O)n_e - N_c^O e^{-h\nu/kT}\right]}{1 + (\tau_u + \tau_\ell)\sigma\bar{I}/h\nu} \tag{11}$$

At zero flux, $\bar{I} = 0$ and α reduces to the linear gain coefficient

$$\alpha_o = \sigma\left[\tau_u(k_3 N_c^O + k_4 N_n^O)n_e - N_c^O e^{-h\nu/kT}\right] \tag{12}$$

Combining this with (11), we obtain the final relationship

$$\alpha = \frac{\alpha_o}{1 + \sigma(\tau_u + \tau_\ell)\overline{I}/h\nu} \quad . \tag{13}$$

We now examine the linear gain, α_o, for pressure dependence. This is a very important parameter since high density storage requires high gas pressures. The pair production cross section σ and level lifetimes are inversely
proportional to the gas density ρ, while N_c^o, N_n^o, and n_e
are proportional to ρ. Consequently α_o is independent
of pressure. The saturation intensity is defined implicitly by Eq. (13) with the value

$$I_s = \frac{h\nu}{\sigma(\tau_u + \tau_\ell)} \quad . \tag{14}$$

This is clearly proportional to the square of the pressure
($I_s \alpha \rho^2$). Therefore, the power stored per unit volume
$P_s = \alpha_o I_s$ is proportional to the square of the pressure,
a very important conclusion as far as increasing the
stored energy density goes.

We can now proceed to examine more quantitatively
the behavior of Eqs. (4) through (7). In Fig. 8, the
stored power density is plotted as a function of time. For
calculational purposes we have used $n_e = 10^{12}$ cm^{-3} at one
atmosphere, and to maintain the same pumping per molecule
we have increased n_e as pressure squared for higher
pressures. Notice that at higher pressures the $V-T$ rates
become dominant after a short time and dump all the energy.
Figure 9 represents the maximum storable energy as a function of pressure (Fig. 8 integrated over time). Thus it is

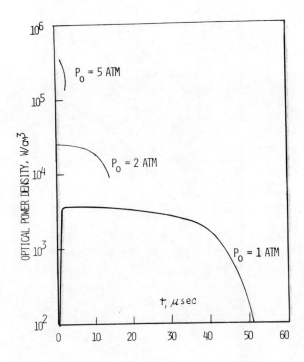

Fig. 8.   Temporal power dependence as a function of
          gas pressure.

evident that although a significant deactivation loss
occurs as pressure is increased, the loss is more than
compensated for by the increase, the volumetric storage
which varies approximately as pressure squared. Finally
we can see the temperature rise as a function of time in
the gas due to V-T processes for various pressures in Fig.
10. Notice the very rapid rise at higher pressures, and
this is another reason why pulses have to be very short at
higher pressures, or else we get into a totally unaccept-
able gain regime as indicated in Fig. 4.

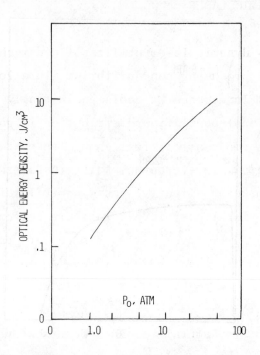

Fig. 9.   Volumetric energy extraction as a function
          of pressure.

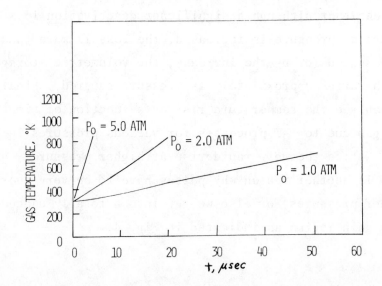

Fig. 10.   Gas temperature rise for various pressures.

5.3. GAS DYNAMIC LASER

The gas dynamic laser utilizes fluid mechanical techniques for producing nonequilibrium vibrational populations.[16-18] In essence it cools an initially hot gas (whose vibrational population distribution is governed by statistical thermodynamics) fast enough that at least some of the vibrational levels cannot maintain Boltzmann equilibrium. To make an effective gas dynamic laser one must then find two vibrational levels that are optically coupled, with the lower level having a much more rapid energy thermalization rate than the upper level. To analyze such a device, one needs to examine the rapid cooling process. One way to cool a gas is to expand it through a Laval nozzle. To understand this process quantitatively, we first examine such a nozzle in the limit of isentropic (adiabatic) flow, which can be done analytically, and then present real gas calculation and results.

The temperature behavior of the gas in such a nozzle,[19-20] is described by the Navier-Stokes equation for velocity

$$\frac{\partial \vec{v}}{\partial t} + \vec{v} \cdot \nabla \vec{v} + \frac{1}{\rho} \nabla P = 0. \tag{15}$$

Taking steady state and performing a line integral along a shear line, we obtain

$$d(v^2/2) + dP/\rho = 0. \tag{16}$$

Combining this with the ideal gas law $P = R\rho T$ and the energy equation $C_p T + \frac{1}{2} v^2$ constant and remembering that $\gamma = C_p/C_v$ and $R = C_p - C_v$ after some manipulation, we obtain $TC_v/\rho R = $ constant. In terms of a "gas stagnation" temperature $T_o \equiv T(v = 0)$ the energy relationship becomes

$$C_p T + \frac{1}{2} v^2 = C_p T_o . \tag{17}$$

With the ideal gas relationship $\dfrac{P}{\rho^\gamma} = \dfrac{P_o}{\rho_o{}^\gamma}$, Eq. (17) may be manipulated into the form

$$\left(\frac{P}{P_o}\right)^{(\gamma-1)/\gamma} = 1 - \left(\frac{\gamma-1}{2}\right)\frac{v^2 \rho_o}{\gamma P_o}$$

$$= 1 - \left(\frac{\gamma-1}{2}\right)\frac{v^2}{a_o{}^2} . \tag{18}$$

We recall that the sound speed $a = a_o = \gamma P_o/\rho_o$ at the stagnation point where $v = 0$. To put Eq. (18) in terms of Mach number $M = v/a$, we multiply and divide its right hand side by a, while remembering that $a^2/a_o^2 = T/T_o$ since $a = \gamma P/\rho = \gamma RT$. We find

$$\frac{P}{P_o} = \left[1 + \left(\frac{\gamma-1}{2}\right) M^2\right]^{-\gamma/(\gamma-1)} \tag{19}$$

and

$$\frac{T}{T_o} = \left[1 + \left(\frac{\gamma-1}{2}\right) M^2\right]^{-1} . \tag{20}$$

We have thus specified how the temperature behaves as a function of velocity or Mach number. We have to further specify the behavior of Mach number in terms of the geometric parameter of the nozzle, namely its area A.

Recognizing that $\frac{dP}{d} = a^2$ if no heat transfer takes place, and combining Eq. (16) with the continuity equation, we find the flow equation

$$\frac{\partial \rho}{\partial t} + \nabla \cdot \rho \vec{v} + \frac{\rho \vec{v}}{A} \cdot \nabla A = 0. \tag{21}$$

In steady state this reduces to

$$\rho VA = \text{constant}. \tag{22}$$

In terms of this we obtain the behavior of velocity as a function of area of a duct or nozzle, namely

$$\frac{dA}{A} = (M^2 - 1) \frac{dv}{v}. \tag{23}$$

If we now specify that at the point where $M = 1$, $a = a_* = v$, i.e., the sonic point, and the associated duct area A_*, with some manipulation we can convert (23) into the relations

$$\frac{dA}{A} = \left[\frac{M^2 - 1}{1 + \frac{1}{2}(\gamma - 1)M^2} \right] \frac{dM}{M} \tag{24a}$$

and

$$\frac{A}{A_*} = \frac{1}{M}\left\{\frac{2}{\gamma+1}\left[1+\frac{1}{2}(\gamma-1)M^2\right]\right\}\frac{\gamma+1}{2(\gamma-1)} . \qquad (24b)$$

We have thus defined the ratio of temperature T to the
stagnation temperature T_O as a function of Mach number,
and the Mach number as a function of the ratio of nozzle
(duct) area A to the area A_* at the sonic line ($M = 1$).
For a hypothetical wedge nozzle the resultant gas temperature as a function of position from the nozzle throat x
is plotted in Fig. 11. Note that at the very early part
of its expansion the gas temperature drops very rapidly,
even for such a noncontoured nozzle. This is exactly what
is needed for freezing of vibrational populations.

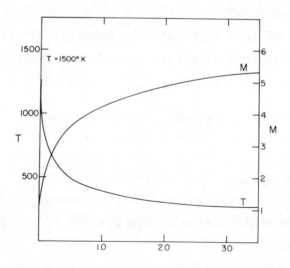

Fig. 11.   *Isentropic temperature and Mach number calculations for wedge nozzle A/A* = 50.*

The vibrational populations are governed by the initial (stagnation) temperature and the associated vibrational energy exchange kinetics that occur as the gas flows down a nozzle. The upper state can be simply described by

$$v \frac{\partial N_u}{\partial x} \simeq - \frac{N_u}{\tau_u} \qquad (25)$$

which states that energy is relaxing from the upper state at an effective rate $1/\tau_u$ which is normally very slow for CO_2[12-14] ($\tau_u \sim 1.5 \times 10^{-4}$ sec for a typical CO_2-N_2-H_2O mixture used in GDLs). Consequently, since the high Mach numbers achieved in the nozzle are due to rapid expansion, very little upper state deactivation occurs, and the upper state population is basically frozen at its stagnation temperature.

The lower state also freezes at the stagnation temperature, but the vibrational energy from this state is dominated by kinetic relaxation processes as described by

$$v \frac{\partial N_\ell}{\partial x} \simeq - \frac{N_\ell}{\tau_\ell} + \frac{N_T}{\tau_\ell} \exp(-h\nu/kT). \qquad (26)$$

Boltzmann equilibrium is approached with respect to the ground state at a very rapid rate[12-14] ($\tau_\ell \sim 5 \times 10^{-6}$ sec for a typical gas mixture). Hence for practical purposes the lower state population is governed not by the stagnation temperature, but by the local gas temperature. Figure 12 shows the behavior of the upper and lower state populations as achieved by a wedge nozzle of Fig. 11. It also shows the small signal gain $\simeq \frac{1}{N_T} (N_u - N_\ell)$. We can see that it goes positive at $x > 1$ cm as the lower level

population drops. Eventually the gain starts to drop off
as the lower level achieves equilibrium with ground state,
while the upper level continues to decay slowly through
collisions with various gas constituents.

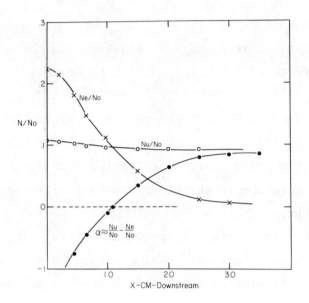

Fig. 12. Population behavior in a wedge nozzle.

Having qualitatively described how a very simple
hypothetical nozzle works, we now examine how a real nozzle is designed and performs. On the assumption that the
gas mixtures chosen have a very slowly decaying upper
$(00^{\circ}1)$ CO_2 state, as per Fig. 12, the gain is determined
primarily by the rate at which the lower level reaches
Boltzmann equilibrium. This rate depends upon the

collisional relaxation time with H_2O as seen in Fig. 13. There we see that the relaxation rate $(1/\tau_\ell)$ is dominated by H_2O, and is relatively slow close to stagnation temperature, but increases very dramatically as the temperature drops, $(1/\tau_{300})/(1/\tau_{1500}) \approx 27$. Consequently, we want to expand the gas very rapidly near the throat, so that the lower state deactivates with the highest rate possible. Consequently, we would use a curved "Laval" type of nozzle whose curvature at the throat is maximized for gain, while keeping the flow from separating. Although a very elegant analytical derivation for a Laval nozzle has been reported by Basov,[21] because viscous effects need to be considered in real nozzles, numerical solutions are normally used.

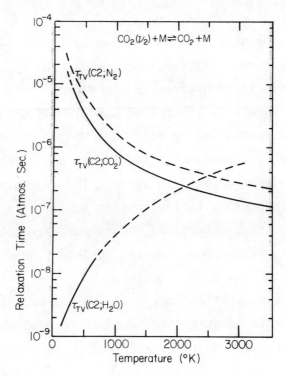

Fig. 13. Lower state relaxation rates.

We start again by writing down the steady state
equations of conservation of mass

$$\frac{\partial(\rho u)}{\partial x} + \frac{\partial(\rho v)}{\partial z} = 0, \tag{27}$$

momentum

$$\rho u \frac{\partial u}{\partial x} + \rho v \frac{\partial v}{\partial z} = -\frac{\partial P}{\partial z} + \frac{\partial \tau}{\partial x}, \tag{28}$$

and energy

$$\rho u C_p \frac{\partial T}{\partial x} + \rho v C_p \frac{\partial t}{\partial z} = \frac{\partial}{\partial x}(Q + u\tau), \tag{29}$$

where τ is the shear stress defined by $\tau = \mu \frac{\partial u}{\partial x}$, where
μ is the friction coefficient and Q is the heat flow.
Here the x axis is transverse to the flow.

These equations are solved numerically while opti-
mizing a wall contour as in Fig. 14. Notice that a certain
boundary layer thickness δ^* results in a real nozzle
which goes to reduce the area ratio. The resulting Mach
number and temperature ratio for such a nozzle is plotted
in Fig. 15. Having determined the temperature behavior in
a real nozzle, we can now compute, in detail, the gain in
power available from such a nozzle.

Using the kinetic diagram of CO_2 molecule in Fig. 1,
we write the rate equations for a laser beam along the
axis (transverse to the flow) as

$$v \frac{\partial N_u}{\partial z} = \frac{N_n}{\tau_{p+}} - \frac{N_u}{\tau_u} - \frac{N_u}{\tau_{p-}} - \frac{\sigma I}{h\nu}(N_u - N_\ell) \tag{30}$$

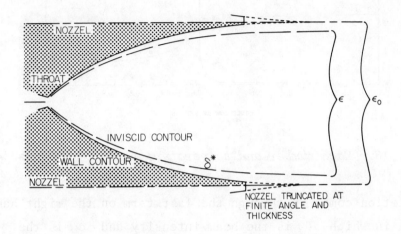

NOZZEL

THROAT

INVISCID CONTOUR

WALL CONTOUR δ^*

NOZZEL

ϵ ϵ_0

NOZZEL TRUNCATED AT
FINITE ANGLE AND
THICKNESS

Fig. 14.   Supersonic nozzle contour.

$$v\frac{\partial N_\ell}{\partial z} = \frac{\sigma I}{h\nu}(N_u - N_\ell) - \frac{N_\ell}{\tau_\ell} + \frac{N_T \exp(-h\nu/kT)}{\tau_\ell} \qquad (31)$$

$$v\frac{\partial N_n}{\partial z} = \frac{N_u}{\tau_{p-}} - \frac{N_n}{\tau_{p+}} \qquad (32)$$

$$\frac{\partial I}{\partial x} = \sigma(N_u - N_\ell)I. \qquad (33)$$

The first equation describes the upper state N_u behavior, i.e., it is being pumped by vibrationally frozen nitrogen N_n, at a rate $1/\tau_{p+}$ and is depleted by backward pumping into nitrogen at $1/\tau_{p-}$ and through collisions into the lower state by $1/\tau_u$. The radiative field

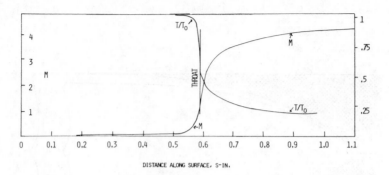

Fig. 15. Mach number and temperature ratio in GDL nozzle.

depletion comes in through the last term on the right hand
side in which I is the beam intensity and σ is the
cross section. The second equation describes the lower
level N_ℓ, which is filled by the radiative term and by
collisions from the upper state, while depleted through its
collisional relaxation time τ_ℓ. The last right hand term
represents the collisional equilibration with ground state.
The third equation represents the pumping of nitrogen from
CO_2 (τ_{p+}), and depletion into CO_2 through (τ_{p-}). Finally,
the last equation represents the laser intensity along the
x axis which is at right angles to the flow and thus along
the beam axis.

In the absence of power extraction, i.e., $I = 0$,
we can describe the small signal gain of our nozzle-GSL-
system. Although the solution is analytic, we only present numerical results in Fig. 16. Gain data is presented
downstream of the nozzle throat at two stagnation temperatures for two different nozzle area ratios. The increase
in efficiency is quite dramatic. One may calculate the
corresponding available vibrational energy, $E = h\nu(N_u - N_\ell)$

for both cases. For nozzles with an area ratio of 24, we
have 4.4 KJ/lb of gas available, and for an area ratio of
56, we have 9 KJ/lb.

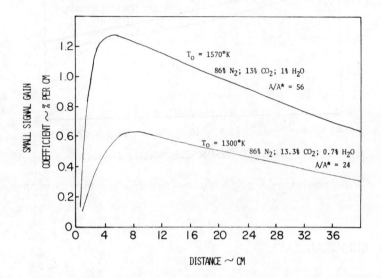

Fig. 16.   Small signal gain coefficient.

The importance of making non-ideal calculations is
shown in Fig. 17. The biggest difference occurs in calculations that involve vibrational relaxation in the flow.
Next in importance is the specification of the boundary
layer growth in the nozzle, a growth which also reduces
gain, since it affects the area ratio of the nozzle and
introduces hot layers of gas (vibrational population non-
frozen) in the flow.

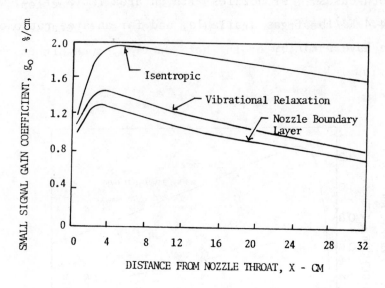

Fig. 17. *Nonisentropic effects on predicted performance.*

5.4. HF CHEMICAL LASER

As distinguished from the gas dynamic laser, the
chemical laser achieves population inversion through chemical reactions that produce reaction products in excited
states, rather than by a quasi mechanical means.[22-24] In
that respect the chemical laser has some similarity to the
electrical CO_2 device. In the latter, there is preferen-
tial pumping of a certain vibrational level by electron
collisions. In the HF laser hydrogen reacts with fluorine
to produce an inversion in some vibrational levels of the
HF molecule.

There are two such reactions between hydrogen and
fluorine. The "cold" reaction takes place between H_2 and
atomic F

$$H_2 + F \rightarrow HF(\nu=i) + H \qquad \Delta h = -31.7 \text{ Kcal/mole,}$$

where Δh is the heat of reaction. The two reaction schemes are presented in Fig. 18. Note that because of larger exothermicity of the hot reaction, much higher vibrational levels of HF are populated.

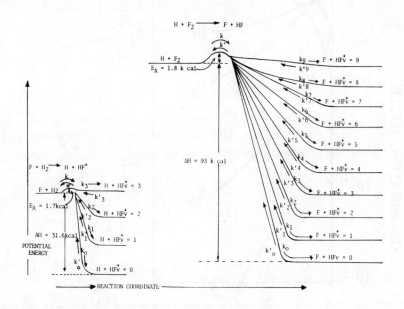

Fig. 18. Reaction diagram of HF laser.

The inversion occurs because some of the reaction rates of Fig. 18 are faster for higher vibrational quantum numbers than for lower ones.[25] Corresponding population densities for various vibrational levels may be achieved as in Fig. 19. Notice that the populations of both the $\nu = 2$ and the $\nu = 1$ levels are inverted with respect to $\nu = 1$ and $\nu = 0$ levels respectively at early positions in a flow where $H_2 + F$ are mixed at $x = 0$. At later

points in the flow, the inversion is lost because of
collisional deactivation of various vibrational levels.[26]

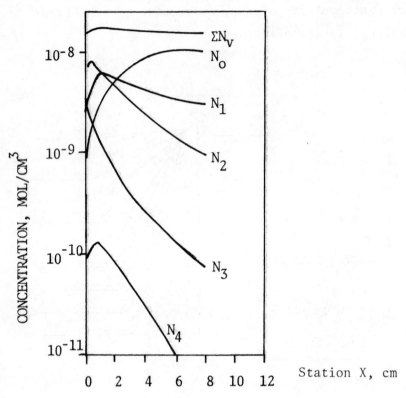

Fig. 19. Calculated excited state concentrations.

The overall diagram of an $H_2 + F_2$ chemical laser
is given in Fig. 20. It consists basically of an $F_2 + D_2$
burner which produces F atoms and DF in thermal equilibrium
and a set of nozzles that drops the temperature of the gas
in exactly the same manner as that of the GDL, but not for
purposes of kinetic freezing. Specifically, since our
source of F atoms is primarily thermal dissociation of F_2,
we need to cool the gas, but since we do not have HF yet,
we do not need to kinetically freeze it. H_2 is then injected into the supersonic flow, where it reacts with the
F atoms as shown in more detail in Fig. 21. Here cold F

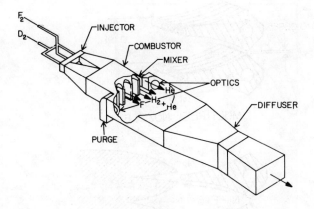

Fig. 20. Representative combustion laser.

atom stream is mixed with cold H_2 in a supersonic channel, where the reaction $H_2 + F \rightarrow HF^* + H$ takes place. Thus, unlike the GDL, no kinetic freezing is needed; on the other hand a more difficult problem exists, namely that supersonic mixing occurs in a chemically-reacting, heat-releasing media. In such a media, gain and optical homogeneity has to be controlled to provide useful optical output.

We now attempt to model such a device following the manner described by Emmanuel[28] in that we assume the reaction

$$F + H_2 \rightarrow HF(\nu) + H \qquad\qquad \nu = 0,1,2,3,\dots \quad (34)$$

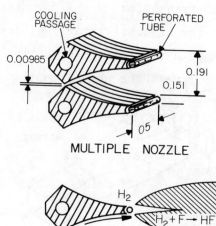

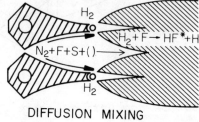

Fig. 21.   *Nozzle diffusion detail.*

is predominant. We can write the population of each vibrational level $n(v)$ in terms of the number of moles of HF
in that particular state

$$\rho v \; \frac{\partial n(0)}{\partial x} \; = \; \chi(0) \; + \; \phi(0)$$

$$\rho v \; \frac{\partial n(1)}{\partial x} \; = \; \chi(1) \; + \; \phi(1) \; - \; \phi(0) \tag{35}$$

$$\rho v \; \frac{\partial n(v_f)}{\partial} \; = \; \chi(v_f) \; - \; \phi(v_f - 1).$$

Here the production rate of the appropriate level by chemical and vibrational exchange means is designated by $\chi(v)$,

the production rate of population is the ν state by
radiative means in the transition $\nu + 1 \rightarrow \nu$ is designated
as $\phi(\nu)$, and ν_f is the highest vibrational level considered. We also denote a flowing system having a velocity
v and density ρ. We invert the above equations to solve
for ϕ as

$$\phi(0) = \rho v \frac{\partial n(0)}{\partial x} - \chi(0)$$

$$\phi(1) = \rho v \frac{\partial}{\partial x} [n(0) + n(1)] - [\chi(0) + \chi(1)] \qquad (36)$$

$$\phi(\nu_f - 1) = \rho v \frac{\partial}{\partial x} [n(0) + \dots n(\nu_f - 1)]$$

$$- [\chi(0) + \dots + \chi(\nu_f - 1)]$$

Summing these equations, we find the production rate

$$\phi = \sum_{\nu=0}^{\nu_f - 1} \phi(\nu) = A_1 - A_2,$$

where

$$A_1 = \rho v \sum_{\nu=0}^{\nu_f - 1} (\nu_f - \nu) \frac{\partial n(\nu)}{\partial x}$$

$$(37)$$

$$A_2 = \sum_{\nu=0}^{\nu_f - 1} (\nu_f - \nu) \chi(\nu).$$

To determine A_1 and A_2, we need to describe the processes which govern the formation of the HF. Generally
speaking, when two compounds (which can undergo a chemical
reaction) are mixed in a flowing system, the chemical reaction will start immediately, i.e., as soon as the reacting
molecules come into contact. The overall rate and spatial
distribution of such a reaction is governed by the chemical
reaction rate and by the rate of mixing. In other words,
the chemical species cannot react until they are mixed or
brought into contact. Since this process is not instantaneous, it, as well as the absolute chemical reaction
rate, governs the formation of HF and consequently power
production.[29]

In order to understand the chemical laser, there are
two limiting cases for the above process that can be examined analytically, In the first case, the mixing is very
fast, and thus the production of HF is limited by the
chemical reaction rate. In the second case, the mixing is
slow compared to the chemical reaction rate, and thus the
power production (production of HF) is governed by the
mixing process. Here we consider the first case, called
"premixed", since it is simpler to treat. It is furthermore associated with much smaller collisional deactivation
losses, a very desirable property for a laser device. One
way of achieving such a situation is to mix the H and F
at very low temperatures. The chemical reaction rate,
because of the exponential temperature dependence, is then
initially very slow, and gases mix without significant
reaction. As mixing progresses and many reacting molecules
come into contact, the slow reaction rate increases due to
the higher gas temperature resulting from the reaction

energy release. Thus HF and power production occur downstream from the mixing, thereby yielding the "premixed"
situation. As mentioned before, such modeling has been
accomplished in a very elegant manner by Emmanuel.[28] G.
Broadwell[30] has extended such an analysis to the mixing
dominated case, whereas Mirels, Hofland, and King[31-32]
have achieved detailed numerical analysis of the realistic
chemical laser, for which both mixing and reaction rates
are important to the power production.

In a steady state oscillator with the optical cavity at right angles to the flow, gain is fixed by the
relation

$$R_1 R_2 \exp [2Lg(\nu, J)] = 1, \tag{38}$$

where g is the gain coefficient per unit length L. The
gain for each P branch vibrational-rotational transition
is given by[27]

$$g(\nu, J) = g_r J e^{-J(J-1)T_r/T} [n(\nu+1) - n(\nu) e^{-2JT_r/T}], \tag{39}$$

where g is a constant proportional to the dipole matrix
element, the molecular weight and density of the species,
and the rotational/translational temperature. For our
purposes we write it as $g_r = C_0 T/T_r^{3/2}$. T is the
translational temperature, T_r is the rotational temperature, and J is the rotational quantum number.

Equations (38) and (39) constitute a set of linear
equations which after some manipulation may yield a solution. Implicit in this analysis are the facts that only

one rotational level for a given vibrational level lases,
and that it is the same J for each vibrational level.
This is normally not far from the real situation in experiments. Solving for $n(v)$, we have

$$
n(v) = \left[\frac{1 - e^{-2J\delta}}{1 - e^{-2J\delta(v_f+1)}} \right] e^{-2J\delta v} n_{tot}
$$

$$
+ \frac{g}{g_r} \frac{\exp[(J^2-J)\delta]}{J(1 - e^{-2J\delta})[1 - \exp[-2J\delta(v_f+1)]]}
$$

$$
\times \left\{ (1 - e^{-2J\delta v}) \left[1 - e^{-2J\delta(v_f+1)} \right] \right. \tag{40}
$$

$$
- v_f e^{-2J\delta v}(1 - e^{-2J\delta})
$$

$$
\left. + e^{-2J\delta(v+1)}\left(1 - e^{-2J\delta v_f} \right) \right\}
$$

$$
v = 0, 1, \ldots, v_f
$$

where $\delta = T_r/T$ and T_r is the characteristic rotational
temperature. Here $\sum\limits_{v=0}^{v_f} n(v) = n_{HF}$, is the total number of
hydrogen fluoride moles per unit mass, a quantity which is
constant in an approximation. Then the x derivative of
Eq. (40) combined with the logarithmic form of Eq. (38)
yields to the definition of A, where during the steady
state lasing process it is assumed that J, a and T are
constant. This is not valid before lasing occurs nor after
cutoff. We find

$$\frac{\partial n(\nu)}{\partial x} = \left[\frac{1 - e^{-2J\delta}}{1 - \exp\left[-2J\delta(\nu_f + 1)\right]}\right] e^{-2J\delta}\, \frac{\partial n_{HF}}{\partial x}$$

and (41)

$$A_1 = \rho v \left[\frac{1 - e^{-2J\delta}}{1 - \exp\left[-2J\delta(\nu_f + 1)\right]}\right] \frac{\partial n_{HF}}{\partial x} \sum_{\nu=0}^{(\nu_f - 1)} (\nu_f - \nu) e^{-2J\delta\nu}.$$

The derivative of n_{HF} has to be determined from the chemical kinetics as well as from the term A_2 which contains both chemical reactions and vibrational energy exchanges. The table below summarizes the important rates. The rates including some energy exchange effects with $\Delta\nu \geq 1$ are plotted vs temperature in Fig. 22.

The distribution constants $a(\nu)$ fix the rate for each vibrational level. Thus, for a particular reaction, the rate into the vibrational level is $a(\nu)k$, where k is the overall reaction constant. The omission of backward rates is accurate only during lasing, while the rate coefficients for $R5$ and $R6$ are only symbolic as they cancel later in the analysis. Without going through a detailed development[28] based on the previous table, it is possible to define $\chi(\nu)$, the net production of excited states, as

$$\chi(\nu) = \rho^2 ka(\nu) n_F n_{H_2}$$

$$+ k_{HF} n_{HF} [a_{HF} - (\nu+1) n(\nu+1) - a_{HF}(\nu) n(\nu)]$$

$$+ k_F n_F [a_F(\nu+1) n(\nu+1) - a_F(\nu) n(\nu)]$$

REACTIONS FOR THE F + H$_2$ LASER [26, 28]

Reaction	Overall Rate Coefficients[a]		Distribution Constants a(v)			
	Forward	Backward	v=0	1	2	3
F+H$_2$ $\rightleftharpoons$ HF(v)+H	$k=1.62\times10^{14}e_1$	$k_b=0$	0.056	0.111	0.555	0.278
HF(v)+HF $\rightleftharpoons$ HF(v-1)+HF	$k_{HF}=6\times10^{16}T^{-1.43}$	$k_b=0$	0	0.167	0.333	0.500
HF(v)+H$_2$(0) $\rightleftharpoons$ HF(v-1)+H$_2$(1)	$k_{H_2}=8.3\times10^5T^{2.2}e_2$	$k_b=0$	0	0.965	0.035	0
HF(v)+F $\rightleftharpoons$ HF(v-1)+F	$k_F=5.4\times10^9T^{1.3}$	$k_b=0$	0	0.167	0.333	0.500
2HF(v) $\rightleftharpoons$ HF(v-1)+HF(v+1)	$k_{fHF}(T)$	$k_b=0$	0	$a_f(1)$	$a_f(2)$	0
2HF(v) $\rightleftharpoons$ HF(v-1)+HF(v+1)	$k_f=0$	$k_{bHF}(T)$	0	$a_b(1)$	$a_b(2)$	0

a

All rate coefficients are in cm^3/mole-sec, and R = 1.987 cal/mole - °K. Here e_1 = exp[-1600/RT] and e_2 = exp[-562/RT].

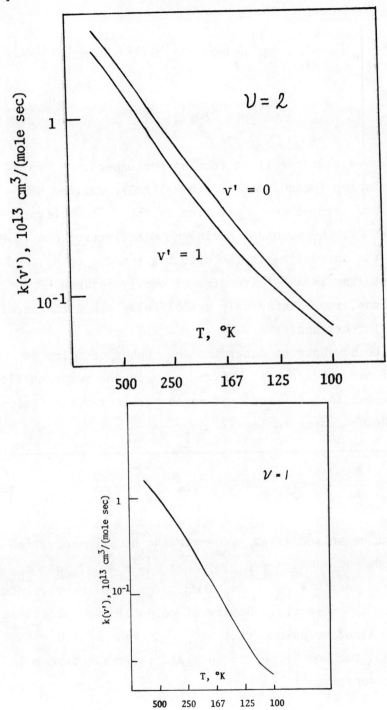

Fig. 22. *Calculated V-T rate coefficients for H +*
          H(ν) → HF(ν) + H.

$$+ k_{H_2} n_{H_2} [a_{H_2}(v+1)n(v+1) - a_{H_2}(v)n(v)]$$

$$\tag{42}$$

$$+ f(k_{fHF}, k_{bHF}) , \qquad\qquad v = 0,1,2.$$

Here we see that the first term of the upper line represents pumping (production of vibrationally excited HF),
the second term of the upper line is the *V-T* deactivation
of HF by HF, the second line is the deactivation due to F
atoms, the third line is the deactivation due to H_2, and
the last line is a *V-V* transfer of energy between HF
collisions, represented only symbolically since it cancels
out in further analysis.

We now have to determine the number of moles of
each of the species n_F, n_{H_2}, n_{HF}, n_H in the reacting flow.
The composition of F and H atoms changes through reaction
1 of the preceding table.

$$v \frac{\partial n_F}{\partial x} = - v \frac{\partial n_H}{\partial x} = - k\rho n_F n_{H_2}. \tag{43}$$

This can be solved if we recognize the atom conservation
relations $n_H + n_{HF} + 2n_{H_2} = n_H^o + n_{HF}^o + 2n_{H_2}^o$, $n_F + n_{HF} = n_F^o + n_{HF}^o$, and $n_F + n_H = n_F^o + n_H^o$. The zero superscripts
indicate the respective number of moles of the species at
$x = 0$. Also, we assume that $n_{HF}^o = 0$ and $n_H^o = 0$. Equation (43) can now be solved to yield the respective moles
of each constituent.

$$\frac{n_F}{n_F^o} = \frac{[1-(n_F^o/n_{H2}^o)]\exp[-k\rho(n_{H_2}^o - n_F^o)x/v]}{[1-(n_F^o/n_{H2}^o)]\exp[-k\rho(n_{H_2}^o - n_F^o)x/v]} \tag{44a}$$

$$\frac{n_{HF}}{n_F^o} = \xi = \frac{1-\exp\left[-k\rho\,(n_{H_2}^o-n_F^o)x/v\right]}{1-(n_F^o/n_{H_2}^o)\exp\left[-k\rho\,(n_{H_2}^o-n_F^o)x/v\right]} \tag{44b}$$

$$\frac{n_{H_2}}{n_F^o} = \frac{n_{H_2}}{n_F^o} - \frac{1-\exp\left[-k\rho\,(n_{H_2}^o-n_F^o)x/v\right]}{1-(n_F^o/n_H^o)\exp\left[-k\rho\,(n_{H_2}^o-n_F^o)x/v\right]}\,. \tag{44c}$$

We can now combine (44b) with (41) to define A_1

$$A_1 = m_1\rho v\,\frac{\partial n_{HF}}{\partial x} \tag{45}$$

$$\tag{46}$$

$$A_1 = m_1 k\rho^2 n_F^o n_{H_2}^o\,(1-\xi)(1-k_1\xi)$$

Here m_1 is a function of rotational and vibrational quantum numbers, temperatures are defined as in (41), and $1/\beta = k\rho\,(n_{H_2}^o - n_F^o)x/v$, $k_1 = n_F^o/n_{H_2}^o$. We can also determine A_2 by substituting Eqs. (42) and (44a, b, c) into Eq. (37). Having obtained A_2, one can now define $\phi_{rad} = A_1 - A_2$ with the value

$$\phi_{rad} = k\rho^2 n_F^o n_{H_2}^o\Bigg\{(m_1-1)(1-\xi)(1-k_1\xi)$$

$$- \left(\frac{\xi}{m_3} + m_5\alpha\right)(1-k_1\xi)\overline{k}_{H_2} \tag{47}$$

$$- k_1\left(\frac{m_2\xi}{m_3}\right) + m_4\alpha\,\left[\overline{k}_{HF}\xi + (1-\xi)\overline{k}_F\right]\Bigg\}\,.$$

Here $\bar{k} = k_{H_2}/k$, $\bar{k}_{HF} = k_{HF}/k$, and $\bar{k}_F/k$; also, $\alpha = (g/g_r)\left(\{\exp[(J^2-J)\delta]\}/Jn_F^o\right)$, while m_2, m_3, m_4, and m_5 are numbers determined by functions of vibrational-rotational quantum numbers and gas temperature.

The input intensity, in watts/cm^2 is given by

$$I_o = 11.96\omega[1 - (R_1R_2)^{1/2}]\phi_{rad}/g \qquad (48a)$$

and the circulating power per unit volume inside the cavity is given by

$$gI_i = hc\mathcal{N}\,\omega\,\phi_{rad}. \qquad (48b)$$

The total output power P is obtained by integration of ϕ along the flow direction,

$$P = hc\mathcal{N}\,\omega\,A\int_o^{x_f}\phi_{rad}\,dx, \qquad (49)$$

where A is the cross sectional area of flow and ω is the wavenumber of the laser transition, h is the Planck's constant, c is the speed of light, and $\mathcal{N}$ is the Avogadro's Number. Note that the intensity increases as the density squared initially, very like the electrical CO_2 case, but soon strong deactivation sets in through thermalizing collisions. This is introduced through in Eq. (47), since g_r is proportional to ρ. Power scales as density, which can readily be ascertained by integrating Eq. (47) until the inverse density dependence of α becomes important.

It is of interest to examine the power per unit
volume available in the laser cavity for three cases of
reacting species. The first case features significantly
more H_2 than F atoms, and $k_1 = 1/3$ was arbitrarily chosen. The second case has exact stoichiometry, and $k_1 = 1$.
The last case corresponds to a mixture lean in H_2, and
$k_1 = 2$. The results are plotted in Fig. 23. They reveal
that when excess H_2 is available, the power per unit volume
generated is very high initially, but it is lost very
rapidly downstream. This is understandable since power is
proportional to the production rate of HF and in a H_2-rich
mixture the production is very rapid. But because the
mixture is rich in H_2, F atoms are consumed very rapidly,
power drops off very dramatically downstream. We can see
further that as stoichiometry is achieved, initial production is slower, but power is available further downstream
as the reaction is slower in consuming F atoms.

The reader should be cautioned to treat the present
analysis as only a qualitative description of the chemical
laser. As was mentioned before, in the real laser, mixing
is always present and cannot be neglected. As mentioned
before, Broadwell[30] developed an analytical model of a
mixing dominated HF laser in an analogous fashion to
Emanuel's[28] premixed model presented here. The assumption
was made that the chemical reaction is instantaneous compared to the mixing rate, and that the mixing zone width,
$\Delta \ell$, grows linearly with x (as it does in turbulent flow).
The derivations result in a ϕ_{rad} as in the premixed case,
except in this case there is only a linear growth with gas
density as opposed to the square dependence of the premixed case:

$$\frac{P}{L h N} = BV N_{\mathrm{F}}^{\mathrm{o}} \rho \left(1 - \frac{\rho}{2\rho_c}\right) E_r.$$ (50)

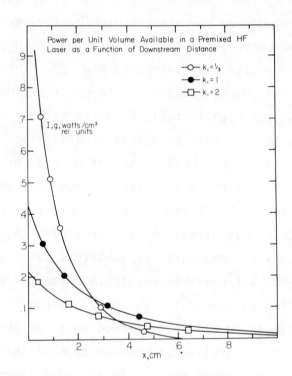

Fig. 23. *Power per unit volume available in a premixed HF laser as a function of downstream distance.*

Here E_r is the heat of the reaction, L is the length, h is the height of the nozzle, N is the number of mixing zones and V is the velocity for growth of the mixing zone. B is a constant having to do with the rotational quantum number J. We see that in such a situation power rises linearly with pressure as in Fig. 24 until a critical value is reached, defined by

$$\rho_c = \frac{DV}{K_{\mathrm{HF}} N_{\mathrm{F}}^{\mathrm{o}}},$$

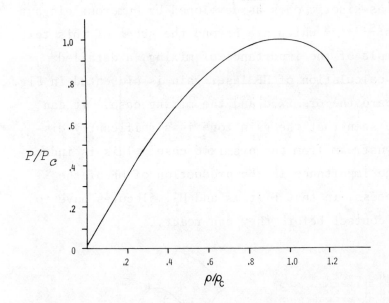

Fig. 24.   *Plot of Eq. (51) showing deactivation coming in*
           at high pressures as the square of the density.

where D is a function of rotational quantum number. At
this point, the second term of Eq. (50) dominates which is
a deactivation term and goes quadratically as pressure.
We can reform Eq. (50) into a dimensionless normalized
equation where $P = P_c$ at $\rho = \rho_o$, namely,

$$\frac{P}{P_c} = 2\,\frac{\rho}{\rho_c}\left(1 - \frac{\rho}{2\rho_c}\right) \tag{51}$$

which is plotted in Fig. 24 and clearly demonstrates the
deactivation coming in at higher pressures as the square
of density.

In the realistic HF laser, mixing processes are as important as kinetic ones as developed by numerous elegant treatments[29,31,32] which are beyond the scope of this text. As an example of the importance of mixing, a detailed numerical calculation of HF laser gain is presented in Fig. 25 to compare the premixed and the mixing case. It can readily be seen that the gain zone is significantly displaced downstream from the premixed case. This is indicative of the importance in the production of HF of the mixing process, in that F atoms and H_2 molecules have to come into contact before they can react.

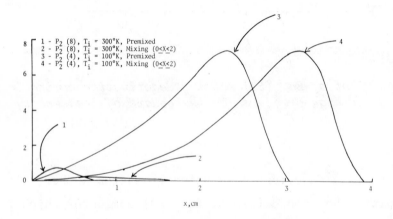

Fig. 25.   HF chemical laser premixed and with mixing option.

REFERENCES

1. J. Wilson, *Appl. Phys. Letters*, **8**, 159 (1966).

2. C. K. N. Patel, *Phys. Rev.* **136**, A1187 (1964).

3. C. K. N. Patel, *Phys. Rev. Letters*, **13**, 617 (1964).

4. C. K. N. Patel, *Appl. Phys. Letters*, **7**, 15 (1965).

5. C. K. N. Patel, *Appl. Phys. Letters*, 7, 290 (1965).

6. C. K. N. Patel, *J. de Chimie Physique*, 1, 82 (1967).

7. C. A. Fenstermacher, M. J. Nutter, J. P. Rink, and K. Boyer, *Bull. Am. Phys. Soc.*, 16, 42 (1971).

8. C. A. Fenstermacher, M. J. Nutter, W. T. Leland, and K. Boyer, *Appl. Phys. Letters* 70, 56 (1972).

9. J. D. Daugherty, E. R. Pugh, and D. H. Douglas-Hamilton, *Bull. Am. Phys. Soc.*, 17, 56 (1972).

10. Englehardt, Phelps and Risk, *Phys. Rev.* 135, No. 6A, p. A1566 (Sept. 64).

11. Phelps, *Rotational and Vibrational Excitation of Molecules by Low Energy Electrons*, Westinghouse Research Laboratories, Scientific Paper 67-1E2-GASES-P2, 1967.

12. Taylor, R. L. and Bitterman, S., *Survey of Vibrational Relaxation Data for Processes Important in the CO_2-N_2 Laser System*, Avco-Everett Research Laboratory Research Report 282 and T89, October and January 1967, respectively.

13. R. L. Taylor and S. Bitterman, *Rev. Mod. Phys.*, 41, 26 (1969).

14. A. D. Wood, unpublished work, Avco-Everett Corporation.

15. N. G. Basov and A. N. Araevskii, *Sov. Phys. JETP*, 17, 1171 (1963).

16. A. R. Kantrowitz, *J. Chem. Phys.*, 14, 150 (1946).

17. V. K. Konyokhov and A. M. Prokhorov, *J. Exp. Theoret. Phys. Letters*, 3, 286 (1966).

18. I. R. Hurle and A. Hertzberg, *Phys. of Fluids*, 1601 (1965).

19. A. M. Kuethe and J. D. Schetzer, *Foundations of Aerodynamics*, John Wiley & Sons, Inc. (1959).

20. J. A. Owczarek, *Fundamentals of Gas Dynamics*, International Textbook Company (1964).

21. N. G. Basov, V. G. Mikhailov, A. N. Araevski, and
    V. A. Shcheglov, *Soviet Physics-Technical Physics*,
    13, 1630 (1969).

22. J. C. Polanyi, *Journal of Chem. Physics*, 34, 344
    (1961).

23. J. C. Polanyi, *Appl. Optics*, 4, Supplement 2, 109
    (1965).

24. D. J. Spencer, T. A. Jacobs, H. Mirels, R. W. F.
    Gross, *Int. J. of Chem. Kinetics*, 1, 493 (1969).

25. J. H. Parker and G. J. Pimentel, *J. of Chem. Physics*,
    63, 1468, (1959).

26. N. Cohen, *A Review of Rate Coefficients for Reactions
    in the H_2-F_2 Laser System*, Aerospace Report #TR-0172
    (2779)-2, Aerospace Corp., Sept. 1971 and references
    therein.

27. G. Emmanuel, *J. Quant., Spectro. Radiative Transf.*,
    11, 1481 (1971).

28. G. Emmanuel and J. S. Whittier, *Closed Form Solution
    to Rate Equations for an $F + H_2$ Laser Oscillator*,
    Aerospace Corp. Report on Contract F04701-71-C-0172,
    (1972).

29. R. Hofland and H. Mirels, *AIAA Journal*, 10, 420 (1972).

30. A. B. Witte, et al., *Aerodynamic Reactive Flow Stu-
    dies of the H_2/F_2 Laser*, AFWL-TR-72-247, Air Force
    Weapons Laboratory, June 1973.

31. H. Mirels, R. Hofland, and W. S. King, *AIAA Paper No.
    72-145*, AIAA 10th Aerospace Sciences Meeting, San
    Diego, 1972.

32. W. S. King and H. Mirels, *AIAA Paper No. 72-146*, AIAA
    10th Aerospace Sciences Meeting, San Diego, 1972.

Part B

CONTROLLED THERMONUCLEAR REACTIONS

SURVEY OF LASER-INITIATED FUSION RESEARCH[*]
Keith Boyer

6.1. INTRODUCTION

The release of thermonuclear energy in a controlled
manner with its promise of providing a relatively clean
and inexhaustible supply of energy is receiving an increasing amount of interest and attention. Shortly after the
laser's invention it was recognized that this device could,
in principle, provide the concentration of energy necessary
to initiate the thermonuclear burning of the appropriate
fuel, but only within a very small volume due to the limi-
tation in total laser energy which might be achieved in a
practical device. However, in order to achieve a sufficient
thermonuclear energy return for the laser energy invested,
it was evident that efficient burning of the fuel would be
required. With these limitations in mind, a study of the

---

[*] Work performed under the auspices of the U.S. Atomic
Energy Commission.

physics of the processes involved led to the concept of
compressing the fuel to high density in an imploding system.

The maturing of this idea over the past ten years
coupled with the development in laser technology and the
experimental and theoretical investigation of the interaction of laser energy with matter has led to the serious
consideration of this concept as an approach parallel to
that of magnetic confinement for the production of electrical energy for utility use by the fusion process. To that
end, substantial programs have been established by the
Atomic Energy Commission at the Los Alamos and Livermore
laboratories with a supporting program at the Sandia Laboratory to investigate the feasibility of this concept.
Smaller programs also exist at the University of Rochester
and at KMS-F at Ann Arbor, Michigan. A large program has
been under way during this period at the Lebedev Institute
in the USSR and at the French Atomic Energy laboratory at
Limeil. More recently, programs have been instituted at
Garching, in West Germany, and at Osaka and Nagoya, in
Japan.

While a favorable outcome of the current programs to
develop this concept is by no means assured, the development
of high intensity, short pulse laser technology and explora-
tion of new areas of physics should prove rewarding in a
practical sense. Of particular interest to the physicist
should be the study of plasmas in the laboratory which are
representative of stellar matter in the core of stars and
the study of nonlinear effects produced by such high densities of radiant energy.

History

Early work on fission weapons at Los Alamos in 1943 by S. Nedermeyer explored the possibility of improving the neutron economy and enhancing the rate of fission energy release by compressing a solid ball of fissile material to high density using a spherical implosion driven by detonating high explosives. This technique did indeed achieve high compressions and as a consequence the technique has been studied and used a great deal since. It is for this reason that the concept of using the laser energy to compress a DT pellet to improve the retention of alpha particle energy and to increase the rate of thermonuclear energy release occurred naturally to workers at Los Alamos and Livermore.

In the early 1960's the possibility of using laser energy to initiate fusion reactions was studied at both Livermore and Los Alamos laboratories. Studies made by Ray Kidder at Livermore including the concept of compression were sufficiently promising that a project was started there in 1963 and a few years later a 12-beam ruby laser was developed to attempt to produce a spherical implosion. In 1960, John Nuckolls, at Livermore, calculated spherical implosions which might be produced by a laser pulse shaped in time and obtained very high predicted compressions. The following year he proposed a thermonuclear engine with a spherical steel containment vessel based on the laser-pellet concept. This work was not part of the laser project directed by Kidder. A study was made of the laser-pellet concept using the implosion technique at Los Alamos in 1961 and a meeting was held to

discuss the advisability of further work, but the state
of laser technology was judged to be inadequate for further work at that time.

In 1962, Basov and Krokhin,[1] in the USSR, showed
analytically that lasers could produce plasmas of the
required temperature to start fusion reactions and
initiated a program which has produced the most advanced
experimental results to date. While they clearly recognized the importance of compression, thére is no evidence
to show that they were aware of the higher densities which
shaped pulses might achieve. They produced neutrons from
laser bombardment[2] in 1968, but recent experiments cast
doubt on the thermal origin of these neutrons.

In 1965, A. Hertzberg and co-workers,[3] at Cornell
Aeronautical Laboratory, made calculations on an imploding
system starting with a preheated low-density gas and later
obtained a patent on the concept.

Numerous other calculations were made of laser-
heated plasmas using various models but not including the
concept of a spherical implosion to obtain high density,
and they all required impractically high laser energies to
achieve scientific breakeven with little hope of giving a
satisfactory net energy return.

In 1969, new programs were started independently at
Los Alamos and Livermore using similar calculational techniques to explore this concept and development work was
started on a variety of new lasers. In 1971, this work
was reviewed by the AEC and the laboratories were encour-
aged to expand this activity. In 1970, the Rochester work
was also accelerated and the KMS program was instituted.

6.2   THERMONUCLEAR BURN PHYSICS

Fusion reaction rates depend on the square of the ion density and increase rapidly with temperature.[4] The most interesting thermonuclear reaction is

$$D + T \rightarrow He^4 + n. \tag{1}$$

There exists an ignition temperature (a few keV for DT) at which the power generation is greater than loss rates, and if reached the temperature rises rapidly to tens of keV, burning the fuel. The percent burn depends on the product ($n\tau$) of the density and time of containment. This is equivalent to the efficiency criterion, familiar from conventional magnetic containment fusion theory. The same concept holds when τ is determined by hydro-dynamic containment, i.e., by the time it takes for a rarefaction wave to move into the center of a sphere of hot fuel, quenching the reaction by cooling it and lowering the density. This leads to a criterion for efficient burn in terms of density and radius,

$$\rho R \sim 1 \ g/cm^2. \tag{2}$$

The burn efficiency is proportional to ρR provided enough energy is generated and deposited to reach the steady burn temperature of tens of keV. The 14-MeV neutrons of Eq. (1) deposit very little of their energy in a sphere of $\rho R = 1 \ g/cm^2$, but the range of the 3-MeV alpha particles is comparable to the dimensions of the fuel. At a ρR of 0.1 g/cm^2 and T of 3 keV, 20% of the alpha energy escapes, but since the range increases with temperature, a greater fraction escapes as the fuel heats. This puts a lower limit on ρR of about 0.2 g/cm^2. The energy necessary to bring the required fuel mass to ignition is then inversely proportional to the density squared

$$E_{IN} = \frac{4\pi}{3} \frac{E_I \, (\rho R)^3}{\rho^2} , \tag{3}$$

where E_I is the ignition energy in J/g. At normal liquid DT density (0.2 g/cm^3) this would require at least 1 g and 3×10^8 J in the fuel for efficient burn. However, if very high compressions (10^3 to 10^4) can be achieved, this energy requirement is reduced to tens of kilojoules, and lower if reduced burn efficiency is acceptable. The DT fusion energy yield is about 10^3 times the ignition energy, and thus one may obtain "scientific" breakeven (E_{out} = incident laser energy) at lower burn efficiencies.

One must consider the efficiency of absorbing the laser energy and of getting it into the fuel. There are a variety of mechanisms and different physical processes of importance depending upon the laser intensity, frequency and pulse duration as well as on the target materials and configuration. When DT burns, it releases about one thousand times the ignition energy per unit mass. However, the efficiency of getting the laser energy into the dense fuel is limited, perhaps to 10% or less, and the fuel burns less than completely, so a yield ratio (thermonuclear output/laser energy) of only about 100 may be expected. In principle, this ratio may be improved if

ρR is sufficiently large to permit absorption of most of the alpha particle energy since part of the reaction energy can be added to laser energy. For a fixed maximum value of density, the burn efficiency decreases with fuel mass, and thus the yield ratio drops off at low mass or low input energy (see Fig. 1). More detailed discussion of these considerations was reported by Nuckolls and Woods at the Montreal Conference on Quantum Electronics last year.

6.3.   LASER ABSORPTION

When intense laser light falls on a solid, even an insulator, the free electrons rapidly cascade and produce an ionized plasma.[5] If the electron density in the plasma is sufficiently high, the light is reflected, as by an ordinary mirror. This occurs where the electron plasma frequency ω_p equals the laser frequency ω

$$\omega_p = \sqrt{\frac{4\pi\, n_e\, e^2}{m_e}} = \frac{2\pi\, c}{\lambda} = \omega. \tag{4}$$

This defines the critical density point for a particular light frequency. This corresponds to 0.15 μ-light (ultraviolet) at solid DT densities, and thus one would expect reflection for all longer wavelengths. However, if there is time for hydrodynamic expansion of the plasma, an "underdense" region where $\omega_p < \omega$ develops (Fig. 2) in which there is collisional absorption (inverse bremsstrahlung). In addition, (Fig. 2) there are many mechanisms which augment this absorption (e.g., resonance

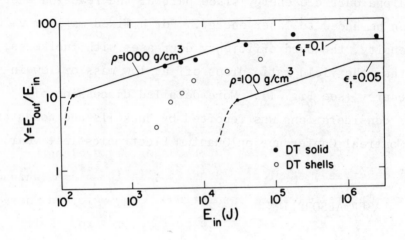

Fig. 1. Yield ratios for DT pellets.

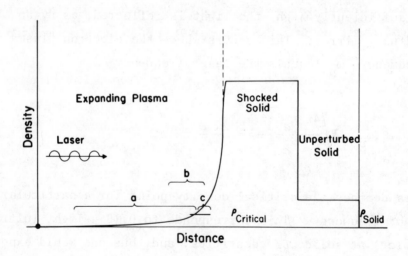

Fig. 2. Laser plasma absorption.

at oblique incidence), produce additional absorption near the critical density (plasma turbulence) or affect the value of ω_p (relativistic effects).

Collisional Absorption

The mass absorption coefficient for this process increases with wavelength, but the shorter wavelength light penetrates to greater densities in the plasma which results in greater total absorption.[6] The absorbed energy goes almost entirely into the electrons, raising their temperature. Coulomb collisions then transfer some of this to the ions in a time given by the ion-electron relaxation rate, which introduces another critical time scale. The absorbed energy can be effective in producing hydrodynamic motion and subsequent ion heating under the proper conditions.

This absorption decreases with increasing electron temperature and increasing laser energy or wavelength because the electron collision time lengthens with in-creasing electron energy. At intensities where collision-al absorption decreases, collective effects referred to as anomalous absorption become important. Here the net absorption is not well known, but it is being studied intensively at this time.

Resonant Absorption

Resonant absorption[7] occurs when the coherent energy is incident at an oblique angle to the critical surface so that a component of the electric field of the wave
is normal to the critical surface where it is resonant with
plasma oscillations. If the electron ion collision frequency is small compared to the wave frequency, these
oscillations build up to large amplitudes. If collisions
limit the amplitude of the oscillations, the electron distribution is thermal. If the collisional effects do not
limit, the oscillations grow until they break in phase
space and very hot electrons are produced.[8]

There is a broad maximum for the absorption as a
function of angle of incidence typically centered about
10° to the normal for cases of interest. As high as 50%
of the incident energy can be absorbed by this process in
favorable cases.

Collisionless Absorption

Collisionless processes, sometimes referred to as
anomalous absorption, start to compete with inverse
bremsstrahlung at intensities of 10^{12} w/cm^2 at wavelengths of 1 μm, and this threshold varies inversely with
the square of the wavelength. This absorption arises from
a large number of instability mechanisms which are predicted by theory and by computer simulations. In general,
they can be divided into three types of processes; electrostatic instabilities, electromagnetic instabilities and
relativistic mechanisms. These have been studied by both

analytical techniques and by use of computer simulation codes. Many experiments are in progress which demonstrate strong anomalous absorption but the multiplicity of mechanisms has made it difficult to identify the effects of each individual instability.

In the neighborhood of the critical surface, the oscillating current flow caused by the electric field of the incident wave can support the growth of longitudinal electrostatic instabilities in the plasma. These have a threshold of 10^{12} to 10^{14} w/cm^2 at 1 μm in a hydrogen plasma which decreases with increasing electron temperature.[9] The most important and most widely studied of these electrostatic instabilities are the two forms of the oscillating two-stream instability,[10,11] the parametric decay instability occurring in an underdense plasma and the modified two-stream instability occurring in an overdense plasma. The effect of these instabilities is to increase the electrical resistivity of the plasma which can result in very strong absorption if the density gradient is not too steep. There is a possibility that this mechanism will produce a small component of very energetic electrons[12] in addition to the thermal distribution.

Electromagnetic instabilities occur when the incident power density is sufficiently great that the $\vec{v} \times \vec{B}$ term in the Lorentz force can no longer be neglected. A typical threshold is 10^{14} w/cm^2 for 1-μm light. The two main cases named in analogy to molecules and solid state processes are stimulated Raman and stimulated Brillouin instabilities.[13] In the former case the incident and reflected light waves interact with plasma oscillations thru the $\vec{v} \times \vec{B}$ force or radiation pressure. The

enhanced backscatter of light occurs about halfway to the
critical surface and at half the frequency of the incident
light. Some heating of the electrons occurs through the
breaking of the plasma wave in phase space. It is not
expected to be a very important process.

        The stimulated Brillouin instability results from a
similar reaction with an ion acoustic wave. It produces
enhanced backscatter at near the incident wavelength and
heats electrons and ions equally. In addition, it can
accelerate some ions to high velocities thereby providing
a possible mechanism for generating nonthermal neutrons.
Apparent agreement between the amount and spectrum of
backscattered light by McCall and co-workers[14] from targets irradiated with 1-μm light at a few $\times 10^{16}$ w/cm^2.

        Above 10^{17} w/cm^2 new phenomena come into play,
especially relativistic effects[15] and radiation pressure.
At very high intensities the electrons are driven each
cycle to velocities near light speed, and there is a maximum current ($n_e ec$) that they can carry. If this is not
sufficient to shield the plasma from the field, the wave
penetrates to greater depths. Direct interaction of the
field with matter by nonlinear mechanisms[16] may produce
strong forces that greatly modify the density gradients
and thus effect the absorption mechanisms already
described.

                        Energy Transport

        The electronic thermal conductivity rises rapidly
with electron temperature ($T_e^{5/2}$) and becomes significant

at $T_e \approx 1$ keV. As long as the electron range is short,
the process can be represented by a diffusion process in
which a thermal wave propagates into the material.[17] The
velocity of the wave front starts out very high and slows
down with time, eventually being affected by hydrodynamic
motion and energy exchange with ions. Whenever the intensity is high, electron conduction must be considered.
There is a limit to the flux which can be conducted even
by hot electrons streaming in a medium, and this can be
reached for high laser intensities. In the region of
critical density the maximum is roughly[12]

$$Q_{max} \frac{w}{cm^2} \approx 2 \times 10^{-8} \, n_c \, T_e^{3/2} \,, \tag{5}$$

where T_e is the electron temperature in keV. If the electron densities are quite low (i.e., at large λ's) and the
energy deposition rate high, the electrons in the absorbing region will become very hot (tens to hundreds of keV).
Nonthermal high energy electrons are also produced by
resonant absorption and plasma turbulent processes. They
will then classically have long mean-free paths and may
not couple their energy to the rest of the electrons and
ions in a useful fashion. This problem is quite complex,
depending upon a variety of factors (geometry and density
distributions), and involves both collisionless and collisional domains, and thus the net effect of hot electrons
is still uncertain. Some leave the system, carrying away
some high energy ions,[18] and possibly a significant fraction of the deposited energy. This expulsion of a small
mass of high energy particles is very inefficient in producing recoil momentum desired to compress the solid.

Where high currents of fast electrons are involved, there
may be collective effects and resistance to flow of the
return currents of cold electrons which might significantly
reduce the range of the electrons compared to the single
particle range. The transport of energy by hot electrons
may help symmetrize implosions, but may hinder them by
preheating of the dense phase, making compression more
difficult.

Having attended to the absorption of laser energy,
although in a less than satisfactory manner, one must
examine the various ways in which this energy can produce
compression and heating of fuel. This is an area which is
open to innovation, invention, and optimization. Most of
the physical phenomena are known at least qualitatively,
but quantitative details must be examined and the practical limitations are not yet defined.

When the laser energy is absorbed forming a plasma,
the plasma ("blowoff") exerts a pressure on the remaining
solid through its particle temperature and its motion.[19,20]
This pressure can be used to effect compression and heating of the remaining fuel (Fig. 3). The time scale is set
by the particle size R, and the speed of sound in the
medium, giving a hydrodynamic time t_h of the order of
nanoseconds at the sizes and temperatures of interest.

If a steady laser intensity I_o is applied to a
plane surface, the plasma expands approximately isothermal-
ly, and the resulting pressure drives a steady shock into
the solid. In a planar case the compression is $(\gamma + 1)/$
$(\gamma - 1) = 4$ for ionized hydrogen with a heat capacity
ration $\gamma = 5/3$. The efficiency of transfer ε_{ks} of
absorbed laser energy into kinetic energy of the shocked

solid is[21]

$$\epsilon_{ks} = \frac{0.04}{\lambda_\mu} \tag{6}$$

where λ_μ = wavelength in microns.

Behind a strong shock the internal energy is equal to the kinetic energy. This would imply a total of 8% efficiency at 1 μm and much less at the CO_2 wavelength of 10 μm, again favoring short wavelengths as did collisional absorption. However, the electron conduction wave can carry energy into the material beyond the critical density and reduce the effect of wavelength. Most of the absorbed energy remains in the expanding plasma. If a sequence of increasing pressures is applied, then a series of shocks pass into the solid multiplying the compression (Fig. 4). The shock speed increases with pressure and in the limit one can think of a continuously varying pressure, sending a series of shocks into a solid such that they coalesce near the center. Each shock multiplies the density caused by the previous shock and a large additional increase in density is produced by the convergence in a spherical system (~ 100 times). The particle trajectories for a spherical implosion including blowoff are illustrated in Fig. 5. The locus of the critical density in the spherically expanding plasma is dependent upon the wavelength. This affects the intensity which in turn determines the extent of anomalous absorption. In order to have the shocks converge at the center, the appropriate laser pulse shape is found to be of the form[22]

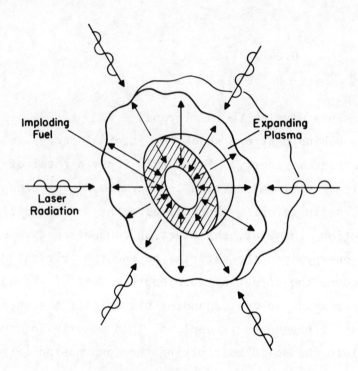

Fig. 3. Pellet implosion.

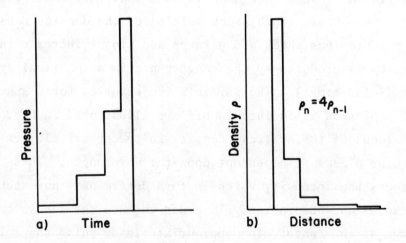

Fig. 4. High density by multiple shocks.

$$\dot{E}(t) = \dot{E}_o \left(1 - \frac{t}{t_f}\right)^{-2} \tag{7}$$

with a cutoff slightly before t_f.

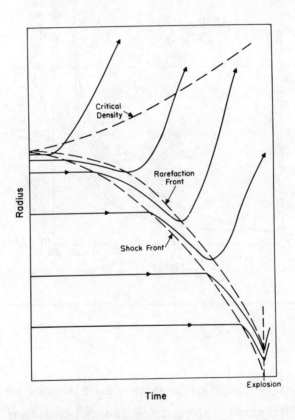

Fig. 5. *Particle trajectories.*

This pulse shape has important implications for laser development and for the interaction regimes of interest. The total pulse length is tens of nanoseconds long, but it terminates in a high power peak tens of picoseconds wide (Fig. 6). The power ranges over several orders of magnitude and therefore includes several interaction modes.

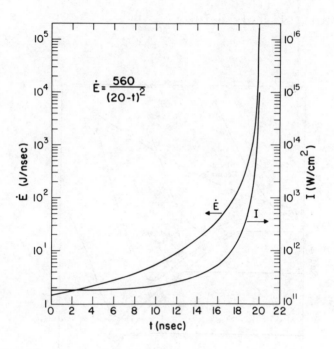

$$\dot{E} = \frac{560}{(20-t)^2}$$

Fig. 6. Laser pulse shape.

This pulse shape or a sequence of shocks heats the material approximately along an adiabat[23] and thus the thermodynamic history of the fuel can be found. The desired final conditions are known from the required ignition temperature, and the density necessary to achieve $\rho R \geq 1$ g/cm^2 for the given fuel mass. This then defines the desired adiabat (Fig. 7), which is reached from the initial conditions by a sequence of two processes. The first strong shock gives the fuel a compression of 4 and a temperature determined by the shock pressure or velocity.

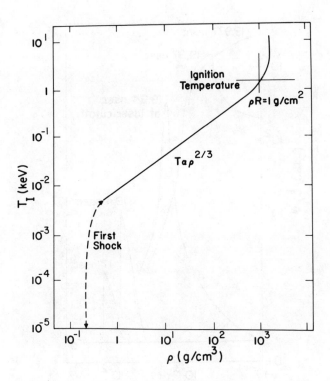

Fig. 7. Fuel implosion adiabat.

Subsequent shocks or increased pressure compress and heat the fuel along an adiabat. The density profile (Fig. 8) develops as a shell of increasing density moving inward toward collapse at the center. At the laser cutoff time the fuel is compressed to a high density (10^2 g/cm^3) and has a large inward velocity (10^7 cm/s). It then coasts in, further compressing and shock heating at collapse. At collapse the fuel is heated to kilovolts as well as compressed to 10^3 g/cm^3 or more.

If the temperature vs density trajectory moves to the left of the ideal adiabat, the fuel ignites at too low a density and causes disassembly before substantial burn

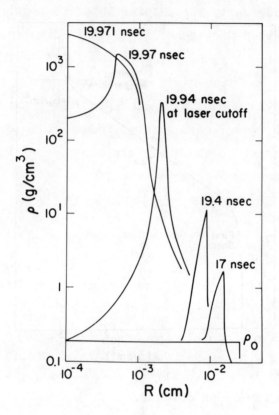

Fig. 8. Imploding pellet densities.

takes place. A small percentage of hot electrons can
cause such an effect, thus giving rise to a concern about
those arising from the various collisionless processes.

A more efficient way to get the energy into the
dense phase is to freely accelerate it like a rocket rather than to shock it.[21] Under steady irradiation of a thin
slab or spherical shell, up to 28% of the absorbed energy
appears as motion of the dense phase, independent of the
laser intensity or wavelength, depending only on the fraction vaporized. Thus a thin spherical shell might be a
better configuration. It allows a longer, lower intensity

pulse to be used, but pulse shaping is still required to achieve the desired high densities. The optimum pulse shape is still to be found for this case. The actual design of pellets and pulses are complicated beyond simple model results by a number of factors including material blowoff, radial convergence effects, nonuniform temperatures and densities in the fuel, nonlocal deposition of laser and thermonuclear energy, etc.

6.4. CURRENT STATUS IN LASER DEVELOPMENT

Two types of laser systems are under development for use in laser-fusion research. One is the Nd:glass laser operating at 1.06 μm, and the other is the CO_2 gas laser operating at 10.6 μm. However, it is generally recognized that neither of these lasers are ideal for this purpose for reasons which will be discussed, so there is a vigorous search under way for new lasers with the desired characteristics.

The Nd:glass laser with a Q-switched oscillator producing a pulse several nanoseconds in duration, is the nearest to an off-the-shelf item. In particular, a 100- to 200-J system with rod amplifiers has been available from the Compagnie General de Electricité (CGE) in France for several years. The largest laser of this type is the nine-beam system built by Prof. Basov's group at the Lebedev Institute in Moscow, which now produces 1 kJ in 2 ns and 1500 J in 30 ns.

Laser systems using rod amplifiers have been operating in the nanosecond region with outputs from 10 to 200 J in laboratories in the United States, England,

France, Germany, Japan, and The Soviet Union for several
years, although most of the target work has been at 30 J
or less because of target-laser isolation problems. A few
of these systems have added, or are adding, disk amplifiers
to extend the available energy, and Faraday rotators or
exploding mirrors to solve the isolation problem, with
several aiming at the 1-kJ region through the use of multiple beams.

Picosecond-pulse lasers have been developed in the
U.S. at the laboratories of Livermore, Los Alamos, NRL,
University of Rochester, and Sandia, but with outputs well
below 100 J on target. Most of these lasers are being augmented by the use of disk amplifiers and multiple beams to
extend their on-target capability into the 1- to 2-kJ region. The most ambitious of these is a 10-kJ system with
ten or more beams being designed at the Lawrence Livermore
Laboratory (LLL) for operation at 100 ps. A much smaller
system is under construction at Los Alamos Scientific Laboratory (LASL) and is scheduled for completion early in
1974, with four beams to operate at 1400 J on target in
250 ps.

The Nd:glass laser system, under development at
LASL, will use four beam paths to generate a total energy
of 1400 joules in 250 picoseconds. This system, as shown
in Fig. 9, will use a mode-locked YAG oscillator, two YAG
amplifiers with 9 mm circular aperture, and a series of
rod amplifiers of Owens-Illinois glass with a maximum aperture of 51 mm. These are followed by disk amplifiers of
51 mm and 85 mm diameter. Faraday rotators with openings
of 85, 51, and 19 mm, and a Pockels Cell of 9 mm aperture
are included for target isolation. One beam path is being

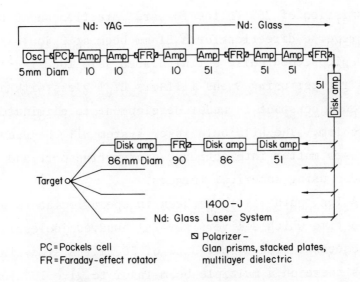

Fig. 9. ND:glass amplifier chain schematic.

assembled and has been checked out through the first 51 mm disk amplifier. The remainder of the first beam path is scheduled for completion by late September. The four beam paths should be operational early next year.

A small system at LASL representing the beam path through the first 51 mm rod has been in operation for some time and is being used on experiments at this time. It provides a good quality beam with 15 to 17 joules on target in 30 picoseconds with a spot size under 50 μm and operates without self-focusing damage at 10 joules on target.

The disk amplifiers are of a modular construction, use edge coating on the Owens-Illinois glass disks which have an elliptical shape to give a circular aperture when mounted at Brewster's angle. Energy storage of 0.5 joules/cm^3 is obtained in the 51 mm disks and 0.4 joules/cm^3 in the 85 mm disks. Faraday rotators have been operated with

a transmission of 75% in the forward direction and 0.003
in the reverse direction for a 51 mm beam at 2 joules/cm^2
in a 30-picosecond pulse but with some self-focusing damage. A rotator using Owens-Illinois EY-1 glass with a
high Verdet constant is under development to eliminate
this problem. The kilojoule laser system will be used to
study laser matter interactions, energy transport and fusion codes using spherical targets.

A long-path laser has been in operation at Livermore
for some time which delivers several hundred joules in a
few nanoseconds with a spot size of 50 μm. A study is in
progress there on a multiple-beam laser to give 10^4 joules
in 100 picoseconds. A Nd:glass laser which can operate at
either a few picoseconds or a few nanoseconds has been in
operation at Sandia for several years. It gives about 35
joules on target. A rod laser system of four beam paths is
also under construction at Sandia with a completion of construction scheduled for the end of this year. It is expected to operate in the few hundred-joule region.

Since peak power is generally limited by self-
focusing in subnanosecond systems, it is advantageous to
extend the pulse length as long as this results in a linear
increase in the available energy, contrary to the formula
for optimum pulse shape. Of course, this is not true for
systems which are energy limited. Therefore, there is a
large difference between the capabilities of a system designed for a given energy output in a nanosecond and one
designed for the same energy in 100 picoseconds.

In general, glass laser systems for laser fusion
research suffer from high cost ($1000/J), low efficiency
(0.1%) and limited power density (10^{10} w/cm^2) due to

destructive self-focusing. Any one of these limitations make such a laser unsuitable for eventual use in a power reactor.

However, these lasers are important tools for use in exploring the interaction physics and in checking the accuracy of the pellet burn codes. The 1400 Joule laser at LASL should be able to attain a few percent of break-even with properly designed pellets while the 10^4 Joule laser at LLL should be able to approach or possibly exceed breakeven.

The only lasers which appear to be capable of meeting the requirements of a power reactor are the electrically-pumped gas lasers, and the only kind of gas laser operating today which might meet these requirements is the CO_2 laser. The "might" includes two reservations: The efficiency achieved is marginal, although ways to improve it are known, and the long wavelength may offer some fundamental limitations, as mentioned later. However, a vigorous search for other lasing media is being pursued with considerable hope of success. Two types of CO_2 lasers have been developed successfully. One type, pioneered in Canada and France, uses photoionization of the lasing medium and a very short pumping time to maintain a large-volume glow discharge at atmospheric pressure. This technique has the advantage of simplicity and low cost for the laser, but the disadvantage of a more expensive and difficult power supply design. It is not known whether this system will work at the pressures and volumes required. The second technique, pioneered at LASL and at AVCO Everett Company independently, uses an electron beam to maintain ionization in the medium and an independently controlled voltage to supply the pump energy.

A CO_2 laser chain with a 1 kJ output in a one nanosecond pulse is undergoing check-out at LASL. This system uses an oscillator of the Lamberton-Pearson type mode-locked by a Brewster-angle acousto-optic modulator to develop a train of 1 ns pulses. One of these pulses is switched out using stacked plates of Germanium mounted at Brewster angles and an AR coated GaAs electro-optic switch driven by a laser triggered spark gap. An output pulse of 1 mJ is obtained with a contrast ratio of 2×10^4. This pulse is amplified by a series of four E-beam controlled electric discharge pumped amplifiers. The final amplifier shown in Fig. 10 has an output circular aperture 25 cm in diameter and it apertures at 3 atmospheres pressure.

An isolation ion cell containing a breakable absorber is used between the second and third amplifiers and a milar film detonated by another laser is placed in a beam moist between the oscillator and the first amplifier. This protects the oscillator from energy reflected from the target.

The first three amplifiers are a meter long and operate with a small signal gain of 5%/cm. The fourth amplifier is two meters long and is designed to operate at 3 atmospheres pressure with a gain of 4.5%/cm. The small signal gain profile is uniform to about 2% over the beam aperture. NaCl single crystal windows are being used presently, but polycrystalline KCl windows are under investigation.

Single line operation of the oscillator has been used to date which extracts about 1/3 of the energy stored in the population inversion in a nanosecond at 3 atmospheres pressure due to the time required for cross relaxation time between the rotational levels. A cold cathode E-beam oscillator operating at 10 atmospheres or higher is being developed to improve the energy extraction and to shorten the pulse length by running on a pressure broadened envelope consisting of many lines.

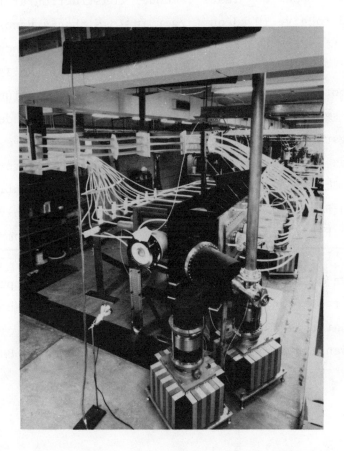

Fig. 10.   1,000 joule amplifier of CO_2 laser system.

Interaction studies have been made using the output of the first three stages on target. Pulse energies up to 10 J in one ns have been used on CD_2 targets to give peak power densities of 5×10^{13} w/cm^2 and this has proved to give similar electron and ion temperatures to that obtained at 5×10^{15} w/cm^2 for 1.06 µm radiation with only a few percent of the energy being reflected.

An 8-beam CO_2 laser is under construction at LASL designed to give 10 kJ on target in less than a nanosecond. This system uses a double sided E-beam amplifier shown in Fig. 11. In order to reduce the complexity of the laser chain, both a two pass and a three pass Cassegrainium Optical system for the final amplifier module is under investigation. Either of these systems will require an isolation cell in front of one of the mirrors to prevent self-oscillation. A possible system of focusing optics is shown in Fig. 12. The final power amplifier assembly is shown in Fig. 13. The performance of this laser compared to the LLL 10 kJ glass laser will depend on how short a pulse can be generated and on how effective the coupling of 10.6 µm radiation to the target proves to be. It should be noted that this CO_2 laser system is about a factor of 10 less expensive per joule and its efficiency should be the order of 7%.

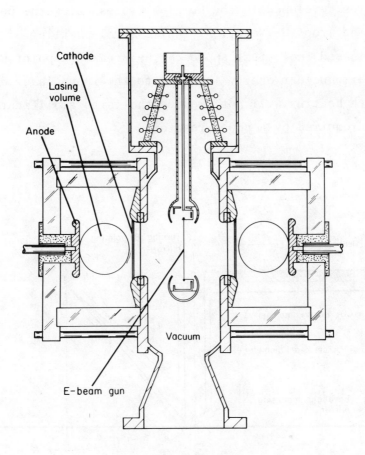

Fig. 11. Double-sided E-beam amplifier.

6.5. REACTOR CONSTRAINTS

The basic concept of laser-initiated fusion involves the compression and heating of the thermonuclear
fuel--a mixture of deuterium and tritium (D + T)--by the
use of concentrated laser radiation. The fuel must be
compressed to a density of about 1000 g/cm^3 and raised to
its ignition temperature of 30 to 40 million degrees centi-
grade to burn a significant fraction of the fuel before the

pressures developed in the burning process blow the pellet
apart and stop the reaction. While simple heating of the
uncompressed fuel might approach the breakeven point where
the thermonuclear energy is equal to the input laser energy, such heating will not produce the large amplification
factor required by a power reactor.

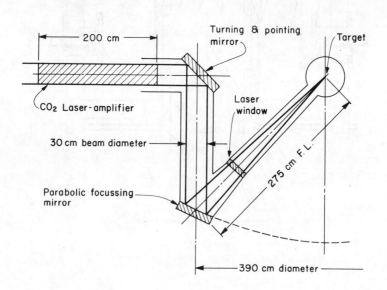

Fig. 12. Schematic of optics for 1250-J amplifier.

The efficiency for generating laser radiation in
short pulses is not likely to exceed 10%, although 20% is
conceivable. The efficiency of CO_2 lasers producing a 1 ns
pulse is about 3 to 4% at this time, but 10% appears to be
a possible upper limit. The efficiency of converting thermal energy into electrical energy would range between 40
and 60% for schemes explored to date, with the lower value

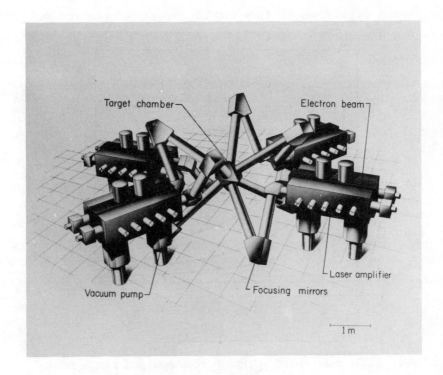

Fig. 13.   10 kJ CO_2 laser system.

being the more probable. To achieve reasonable plant in-
vestment costs, a power plant should have a circulating
power (primarily the electrical power furnished to the laser in this case) amounting to less than 30% of the electrical power generated. As shown in Fig. 14, this requires
an amplification factor of at least 50 for an economically
competitive power plant.

Calculations of the dynamics involved in compressing and heating a pellet by laser radiation show that only
10% or less of the laser energy absorbed by the pellet is
transferred to the fuel. The rest of the energy goes into
blowoff material or is used up in heating and compressing

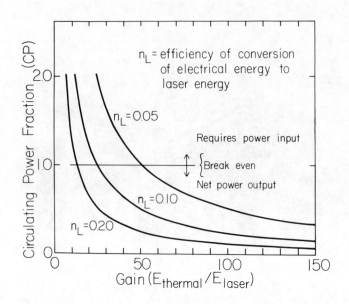

Fig. 14. *LCTR circulating power; energy balance break-even point is indicated for various energy conversion efficiencies.*

material that does not burn. The energy produced by complete burning of the thermonuclear fuel is about 1000 times
the energy invested in the fuel to establish ignition conditions. In principle, amplification factors in excess of
100 should be possible for the following reasons: The energy needed to compress the fuel is less than the energy
required to heat the fuel to the ignition temperature.
Therefore, it seems plausible that only the center of the
compressed sphere needs to be heated to the ignition temperature when the resultant burn should propagate outward.
While calculations indeed predict this type of propagation,
it has not yet been possible to calculate amplification
factors much in excess of 100.

The laser pulse should be strongly varying with time, as discussed elsewhere,[24] with one half of the energy being delivered in the last 100 ps for a solid DT pellet and a 100 kJ pulse. To some extent this requirement can be softened by pellet design. For instance, a hollow DT shell is predicted to work well, with the pulse intensity increasing linearly with time over a period of 1 ns. However, such shells may not implode symmetrically, particularly if the ratio of the shell's radius to its thickness is too high or if the laser radiation is not sufficiently uniform. One-dimensional calculations, in which the radius and density are expanded in spherical harmonics, show this effect clearly in Fig. 15, where $\ell = 1$ indicates illumination from one direction, $\ell = 2$ from two, etc., and P_1

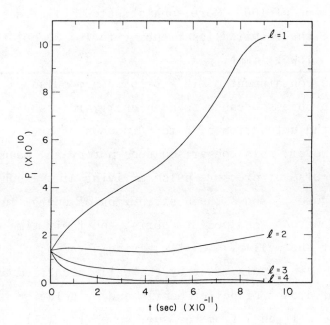

Fig. 15.   *Effects on implosion symmetry of number of illumination sources.*

is the departure of the pressure distribution from spherical symmetry.

The laser energy required for a power reactor of
this type will, of course, depend strongly on laser performance and pellet design as shown in Fig. 16. It assumes
idealized performance of a solid sphere of DT without any
allowance for non-Maxwellian distribution of electron energies due to the absorption process, for the lack of symmetry of the implosion, or the departure from optimum
pulse shape. The line labeled Pellet X in Fig. 16 represents a hypothetical design in which the maximum efficiency of coupling the absorbed energy to the fuel is somehow
achieved. In practice, these assumptions will probably
not be realized, so that the true economic threshold for
such a reactor may require a laser energy of 10^6 J with an
amplification of 100. More sophisticated pellet design
may reduce the required laser energy to 10^5 J, but this is
probably a lower limit.

The containment of 10^7 to 10^8 J per pulse raises
numerous problems because such an energy release is equivalent to the detonation of 5 to 50 pounds of high explosive. However, this comparison does not by any means apply
to the impulse or pressure pulse arriving at the containing
wall. Figure 17 shows the distribution of energy in
x-rays, neutrons, and pellet debris, and their time of
arrival at the wall of a cavity having a radius of one meter. The main impulse felt by the wall is carried by a
very small amount of pellet debris and by ablation or
evaporation (if any) from the surface of the wall. The
neutrons are absorbed in the lithium blanket behind the

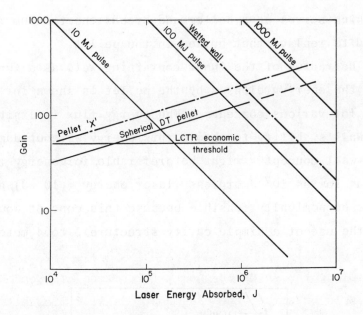

Fig. 16. *Overall design constraints of laser-controlled thermonuclear reactor.*

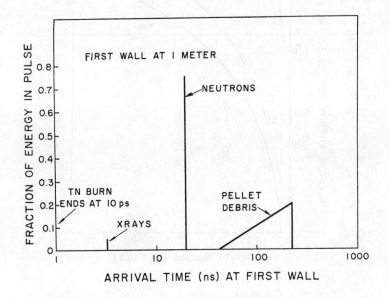

Fig. 17. *Timescale of energy incident on LCTR first wall.*

wall, which serves as a boiler and breeds the tritium
required to replace that burned in the pellet.

The radius of the inner containing wall as a function of the energy released by the pellet is shown in
Fig. 18 for various concepts. The energy flux is limited
by the wall's ability to absorb this energy without damage.
The dry-wall concept[25] might be preferable for energy releases as low as 10^7 J or less (laser energy = 10^5 J) and
might be economically feasible because this concept would
permit the use of a simple cavity structure 3 to 4 meters

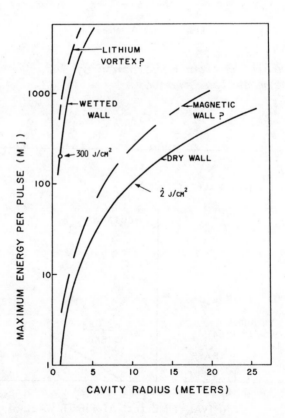

Fig. 18. Effect of pulse energy on cavity radius of a
          LCTR.

in radius. However, a wetted-wall design[26] with its much higher permissible energy flux would be needed for higher thresholds. While the lithium vortex, proposed by A. Fraas[27] of Oak Ridge National Laboratory, has the highest flux capacity, it is difficult to illuminate the target from more than one direction. However, if pellets of satisfactory design could be developed for such illumination, the vortex might prove to be a satisfactory approach.

A major design problem is that of maintaining optical integrity in a reactor system. The optical surfaces transporting the beam must be protected to some extent from pellet debris and from x-rays; however, because x-rays are absorbed much more strongly than laser radiation, the allowable x-ray flux will be much less. Figure 19 shows the ratio of x-ray flux to laser flux that is permissible on the last optical surface as a function of f-number of the optical system. Assuming a pellet gain or amplification factor of 100 and a total laser energy of 10^6 J, the various curves correspond to the number of beams (N_B) used to heat the pellet. The horizontal lines give the various focal lengths in meters. In addition to the damage to optical surfaces, the refraction of the beam by the low-pressure lithium vapor must also be considered for concepts other than the dry wall. As shown in Fig. 20, the allowable lithium vapor pressure ranges between 1 and 0.1 Torr, depending on target size.

While none of the above considerations are absolute-- present lack of knowledge of design and operating conditions offers considerable latitude--these considerations may still define qualitative boundary conditions that have to be considered in any laser-fusion reactor design.

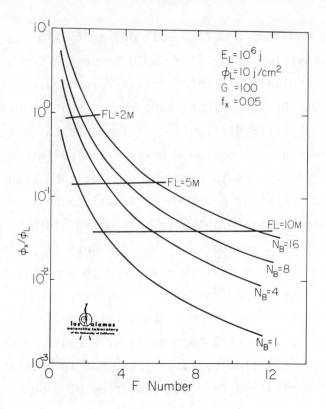

Fig. 19.   LCTR optical system parameters.

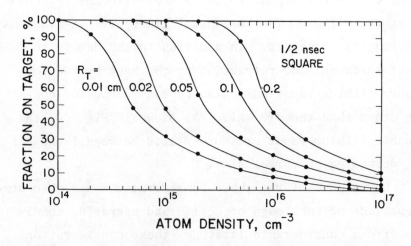

*Fig. 20.   Fraction on target as a function of atom density
for various target sizes.*

REFERENCES

1. N. G. Basov and O. N. Krokhin, English Translation, *Soviet Physics JETP* <u>19</u>, 123 (1964).

2. N. G. Basov, et al., English Translation, *JETP Letters* <u>8</u>, 14 (1968).

3. J. W. Daiber, A. Hertzberg and E. E. Wittliff, *Phys. Fluids* <u>9</u>, 617 (1966).

4. David J. Rose and Melville Clark, Jr., *Plasmas and Controlled Fusion*, page 82, MIT Press and John Wiley, New York (1961).

5. A. Caruso, et al., *Il Nuovo Cimento 45B*, 176 (1966).

6. R. Cooper, "Collisional Heating in an Expanding Plasma," to be published in the *Bulletin of the American Physical Society*.

7. R. P. Godwin, *Phys. Rev. Letters* <u>28</u>, 85 (1972).

8. J. P. Freidberg, R. Mitchell, R. Morse and L. Rudsinski, *Phys. Rev. Letters*, <u>28</u>, 795 (1972).

9. N. Nishikawa, *J. Phys. Soc. Japan* <u>24</u>, 916 (1968).

10. J. P. Freidberg and B. M. Marder, *Phys. Rev. A* <u>4</u>, 1549 (1968).

11. W. L. Kruer and J. M. Dawson, *Phys. of Fluids* <u>15</u>, 446 (1972).

12. R. L. Morse and C. W. Nielson, "Occurrence of High Energy Electrons and Surface Expansion in Radiantly Heated Target Plasmas," Los Alamos Scientific Laboratory Report, LA-4986-MS, to be published in *Physics of Fluids*.

13. D. W. Forslund, J. M. Kindel and E. L. Lindman, *Phys. Rev. Letters* <u>29</u>, 249 (1972).

14. G. H. McCall, R. P. Godwin and J. F. Kephart, "Measured Polarization of X-rays from Laser Produced Plasmas," to be published in the *Bulletin of the American Physical Society*.

15. Kaw and J. Dawson, *Phys. of Fluids* 13, 472 (1970).

16. H. Hora, *Non-linear Forces in Laser Produced Plasmas in Laser Interaction and Related Plasma Phenomena*, Vol. 2, page 341, ed. by H. J. Schwartz and H. Hora, Plenum Press, New York (1972).

17. R. C. Mjolsness and H. M. Ruppel, *Phys. of Fluids* 15, 1620 (1972).

18. A. V. Gurevich, et al., *JETP* (English Trans.) 22, 449 (1966).

19. Y. V. Afanasyev, O. N. Krokhin, and G. V. Sklizkov, *IEEE J. Quantum Electronics*, QE2, 483 (1966).

20. C. Fauquignon and F. Floux, *Phys. of Fluids* 13, 386 (1970).

21. R. Cooper, "Motion of Solid D_2 under Laser Irradiation," *AIAA Paper* 72-721 (1972).

22. S. Clark, *Bulletin of the American Physical Society*, 17, 1035 (1972).

23. C. Evans and F. Evans, *J. Fluid Mech.* 1, 399 (1956).

24. K. Boyer, *Astronautics and Aeronautics*, Vol. II, No. 1, 28 (1973).

25. B. Freeman, L. Wood, J. Nuckolls, "Some General Design Considerations Regarding Laser-Fusion CTR Power Plants," University of California Lawrence Livermore Laboratory, Livermore, California (1971).

26. L. A. Booth, *Nucl. Eng. and Design* 24, 263 (1973).

27. A. P. Fraas, "The Blascon--An Exploding Pellet Fusion Reactor," *Oak Ridge National Laboratory Report ORNL-TM-3231* (1971).

LASERS FOR FUSION

John R. Murray and Paul W. Hoff

7.1. INTRODUCTION

Significant energy yield from thermonuclear fusion
of a small, inertially confined, deuterium-tritium pellet
requires an energy delivered to the pellet of some 10^4 -
10^6 joules in 10^{-9} - 10^{-10} sec, as discussed in more detail
by Keith Boyer and Richard Morse in Chaps. 6 and 8 respectively.[1] Large lasers concentrate energy very effectively
in space and in time and are currently the best tools
available for such experiments.

In this chapter we give a brief overview of the
state-of-the-art in laser systems suitable for concentrating large energies on a small thermonuclear target.
Section 7.2 discusses the general design parameters of
high energy subnanosecond-pulse laser amplifiers. Section
7.3 compares several laser transitions with these requirements and discusses the performance of several lasers now
operating or projected for the next few years. Sections
7.4 and 7.5 discuss excimer lasers and a quadrupole

transition gas laser, both of which may prove more suitable for practical applications of laser fusion than existing lasers. Section 7.6 treats the more speculative
possibility of laser amplifiers operating on multi-quantum
transitions.

7.2. DESIGN PARAMETERS OF A LASER FOR FUSION

The design of any specific laser system for high
energy short pulses is complex and requires compromises to
work around the limitations of whatever particular laser
transition and materials may be involved. Some rather
general limitations and desirable properties for such lasers can be identified, however, and these features can
then be used to judge the potential of present lasers or
of any proposed new lasers for fusion research and to
guide the development of lasers for fusion or for other
short pulse applications.

Limits On Maximum Energy Flux And Intensity

Solids. Damage to optical components and to solid
laser materials from non-linear optical effects and breakdown limits the allowable intensity flux and energy flux in
a laser amplifier. A recent review by A. J. Glass and
A. H. Guenther[2] discusses the various damage mechanisms in
some detail.

We summarize the most important limitations in
Table 1. Self-focusing[3] is not in itself damaging but
produces high intensities and consequent avalanche

TABLE 1

SUBNANOSECOND-PULSE DAMAGE THRESHOLDS OF OPTICAL MATERIALS

	Dependence (for a subnanosecond pulse)	Threshold ($\lambda \sim 1\ \mu m$)
Electron avalanche breakdown		
bulk	ε	$10\text{-}100^+$ j/cm^2
surface	ε	1-10 j/cm^2
Thin films (dielectric mirrors, etc.)	ε	~ 3 j/cm^2
Self-focusing (and consequent break-down)	$I,\ \ell,\ \dfrac{\delta I}{\delta r}$	$\sim 10^{10}\text{-}10^{11}$ w/cm^2 (for present solid-state amplifier designs) [1-10 j/cm^2 in 100 psec]

ε = energy flux; I = intensity; ℓ = propagation distance through the nonlinear material; $\dfrac{\delta I}{\delta r}$ = rate of change of the intensity across the amplifier aperture (transverse to the beam propagation direction).

Note that the $\dfrac{\delta I}{\delta r}$ dependence puts strict limits on such perturbations as diffraction from apertures and dust spots in a laser amplifier for which I and ℓ are near the self-focusing limit. Usually this is the case in neodymium glass amplifiers. For more detail on the behavior of self-focusing see the papers listed in Ref. 2.

breakdown, as well as a loss of beam quality. Gross de-
fects in optical materials, such as bulk inclusions in laser crystals or optically absorbing impurities in windows,
are neglected. The threshold values given in the table
are order of magnitude values for lasers of wavelength
near one micron. Data indicate that the damage threshold
decreases at λ = 0.69 μm relative to 1.06 μm for pulses of
a few nanoseconds duration[4], but the complete wavelength
dependence of damage is not too well understood. For our
purposes it is sufficient to say that a practical laser
amplifier at $\lambda \simeq$ 1 μm will be limited to a few joules/cm^2
of output window area to avoid damage to optical components
or the laser medium. The permissible flux may be increased
somewhat by operation at shorter wavelengths or by improved
materials processing techniques (particularly surface finishing techniques) but is unlikely to go above a few tens
of joules/cm^2.

There is less information available on nanosecond-
pulse damage phenomena at much longer wavelengths such as
the 10.6 μm CO_2 laser. Surface damage thresholds[5] for
pulses of a few nanoseconds in materials such as NaCℓ appear to be 2-5 j/cm^2, or about the same as at 1 μm. It
is at present more difficult to fabricate high quality
surfaces on materials such as NaCℓ which are transparent in
the medium infrared than it is to fabricate near infrared
and visible components.

At wavelengths very much shorter than 1 μm, damage
thresholds decrease. The damage mechanisms noted so far
have ignored intrinsic optical absorption and the thermal
stress, enhanced electron avalanche breakdown, and optical
nonlinearities resulting from it. All optical materials

are opaque at $\lambda < 0.1$ μm and most convenient materials absorb strongly at 0.15 μm, so wavelengths this short are not suitable for high energy lasers unless a windowless configuration is developed. The intensity in a short, high energy pulse in these lasers is high enough that two-quantum absorption becomes an important effect: a crude estimate[6] indicates that the two-quantum absorption of, for example, the 0.17 μm Xe_2^* excimer laser in crystals such as LiF or MgF_2 might reach ~ 3 cm^{-2} at an intensity of 10^{10} w/cm^2. A laser with output intensities of this magnitude is therefore restricted to wavelengths longer than 0.3 μm.

Two-quantum absorptions can also be important in other lasers. A recent measurement of a neodymium glass indicates considerable two-photon absorption in Nd^{3+} ion levels.[7] In this case, however, the absorption may be an advantage since it limits self-focusing.

Gases. Components for gas lasers of course suffer the same limitations as those for solid state lasers, but the active medium is at a much lower particle density and this causes some differences. Self-focusing can probably be neglected[8] in gases at any pressure likely to be useful in a gas laser, unless the lasing species appears in very high concentration. Electron avalanche breakdown in gases is an energy dependent effect for long wavelengths and is proportional to $\frac{\lambda^2}{p}$ where p is the gas pressure. A typical CO_2-N_2-He laser gas mixture with some pre-existing ionization breaks down with a visible spark at ~ 10 j/cm^2 at atmospheric pressure and $\lambda = 10.6$ μm.[9] There is also a strong thermal self-defocusing effect at energies above ~ 3 j/cm^2 under these conditions.[10] High pressure CO_2 amplifiers may be limited by gas breakdown but it is not

likely to be important at shorter wavelengths. At considerably shorter wavelengths, however, multi-quantum ionization and other effects may again lower the threshold for
breakdown. Note that consequences of an accidental breakdown in a gas laser are less serious than in solid lasers
which suffer permanent damage.

Efficient Energy Extraction In An Amplifier

Energy is extracted efficiently from an inverted laser transition only when the energy flux in the amplifier
exceeds the energy flux required to saturate the transition. For a photon energy $h\nu$ and stimulated emission
cross section σ, the saturation energy flux is $\frac{h\nu}{\sigma}$ for
a wide variety of circumstances and is so defined here.[11]
If the upper laser level is repopulated during the pulse,
the saturation energy flux for a given transition is increased; however, this is seldom significant in a 10^{-9} -
10^{-10} sec pulse. Energy extraction in such short pulses is
limited to the instantaneous value of the energy stored in
the laser population inversion.

The stimulated emission cross section σ is given
by

$$\sigma(\nu) = \frac{\lambda^2}{8\pi} \frac{g(\nu)}{\tau_r} ,$$

where τ_r is the radiative lifetime and $g(\nu)$ the lineshape (normalized to unity) of the laser transition. The
small-signal intensity gain per unit length of the laser

active medium is $\sigma(\nu)\ \Delta N$ where ΔN is the population
inversion or $h\nu\ \Delta N$ is the energy stored per unit volume.

The shape of a pulse propagating through a saturated
amplifier is distorted when the energy flux in the pulse
exceeds the saturation flux of the amplifier. In general
the risetime of the pulse is shortened, the fall time
lengthened, and small perturbations on the input intensity
distribution can become rather large perturbations on the
output distribution. The exact details of the pulse shape
can become quite complex. To avoid these effects the flux
in a practical amplifier will probably be limited to less
than a few times the saturation flux.

Energy fluxes below the saturation flux give linear
amplification, but the energy extraction efficiency is reduced. Since it is much easier to carefully shape a low
energy pulse than a pulse at 10^4 - 10^6 joules, it is likely that initial studies of laser fusion with carefully
tailored pulses (see Chap. 8 by R. Morse) will use linear
rather than saturated amplifiers. For any applications
which require high efficiency, however, a saturated final
amplifier will be required.

Inversion Lifetime In The Amplifier

Nonradiative decay processes and spontaneous fluorescence of the laser transition limit the length of time
for which a population inversion can be maintained in a
laser amplifier. An amplifier is efficient only if the
time required to establish the population inversion is less
than the inversion lifetime. It is fairly easy to transfer
the electrical energy required to pump a 10^4 - 10^6 joule

laser of reasonable volume in milliseconds and barely possible to transfer it in somewhat less than a microsecond.
If such energies could be transferred to small volumes in
a nanosecond, there would be much less interest in lasers
for fusion. We might summarize that a millisecond inversion lifetime in the amplifier is desired, but a microsecond lifetime is acceptable.

Limits On Amplifier Size And Energy Storage From Superfluorescence And Parasitics

Spontaneous fluorescence of the laser transition is
amplified with the small-signal gain of the laser medium as
it propagates out of the amplifier. This "superfluorescence" is a mechanism which increases the effective radiative rate and shortens the inversion lifetime in the amplifier. The decrease in the inversion lifetime depends
on the geometry of the amplifier, but as a rule of thumb[12]
superfluorescence is significant (and minimizing it strongly influences amplifier design) when the small signal gain
$\sigma \Delta N \ell$ across the amplifier is greater than 5. The energy
stored in the amplifier is proportional to the population
inversion per unit volume ΔN and to the volume of the
amplifier, which is $\sim \ell^3$. The rate of energy loss from
superfluorescence is proportional to $r\sigma \Delta N \ell$, where r is
the rate of spontaneous emission on the laser transition;
however, r is also proportional to σ so the superfluorescent loss rate varies as $\sigma^2 \Delta N \ell$. Clearly, σ should be
as small as possible in a high energy storage amplifier.
Stray reflections or scattering may provide enough
feedback into an amplifier for superfluorescence to become

an actual parasitic oscillation which destroys the population inversion. These spurious oscillations are also much
more easily designed out of a high energy storage amplifier
if σ is small.

As these remarks show, superfluorescent and parasitic losses scale up with the size and energy storage of the
amplifier. Since multiple laser beams must be used to
illuminate a fusion target to achieve symmetrical compression in any case, (and also fabrication of optics is very
much more difficult in large sizes), lasers for fusion experiments will have multiple parallel final amplifiers,
rather than a single amplifier capable of delivering the
entire pulse energy.

Amplifier Staging And Isolation

A high energy 10^{-10} sec pulse cannot be generated in
a large laser amplifier with current technology, so any
lasers for fusion in the near future will require a low
energy mode-locked oscillator followed by a chain of amplifiers increasing in aperture and volume to increase the
pulse energy to the final value required. The energy gain
from oscillator to output pulse in such a system will be
$\sim e^{10}$ to e^{16}. Superfluorescent and parasitic losses can
therefore be quite serious and the amplifier stages must be
carefully isolated to reduce them. Isolation in present
high energy amplifiers is usually geometrical: stages are
spaced far enough apart that the intensity of the highly
divergent superfluorescence from a stage of the amplifier,
which falls into the input aperture of the next stage, is

within tolerable limits. The laser pulse is collimated and is not affected by the long propagation distances except for a small diffraction correction.

At low pulse energies, Kerr or Pockels Effect electro-optic shutters can be used for isolation, but electro-optic shutters cannot presently be made with a large enough aperture to be useful in a high energy amplifier. Typical samples of nonlinear materials also have rather lower damage thresholds than laser glass or passive optical elements[2], possibly because the material is not of high quality.

A saturable absorption cell may be used to isolate stages in a large laser and such isolators are being carefully studied. Typical organic-dye-in-solvent absorbers, such as are commonly used at low energies in ruby and neodymium glass lasers, do not appear to be suitable for high energy applications. The solvents in such absorbers have large optical nonlinearities and cause strong self-focusing. Absorbing gases have been used with CO_2 lasers with some success, but further development is clearly needed.

Saturable absorbers distort the envelope of transmitted pulses. They will not be suitable isolators in lasers used for experiments requiring careful pulse tailoring unless the distortion can be compensated or fortuitously happens to give an appropriate pulse shape at the output.

The ideal application of a saturable absorber is to add a small concentration of absorbers to the laser active medium so that the small signal gain in the amplifier is reduced or even made less than zero. Superfluorescence can then no longer limit the size or inversion density of an

amplifier. Such an absorber would presumably be an ion
doped into neodymium glass with a strong absorption at
1.06 μm, or a molecule introduced into the gaseous active
media of the CO_2 or other gas lasers which absorbs strongly
at the laser wavelength. The absorber must also, of course,
not affect the kinetics of the population inversion.

The conditions which a saturable absorber must satisfy to be useful in a high energy isolator (either discrete or combined in the amplifier) are

$$\sigma_{absorber} \geq 10\sigma_{laser}$$

$$\tau_r > \tau_{absorber} > \tau_{pulse}$$

The large cross section for the absorber implies a small
saturation energy and consequently a small loss of energy
in opening the isolator with the leading edge of the laser
pulse. The radiative lifetime of the laser gain medium
(suitably shortened by superfluorescence) must be longer
and the pulse length shorter than the relaxation time of
the absorber so that the absorber will be saturated by the
pulse, but not by fluorescence.

Target Reflections

Some fraction of the laser energy incident on a
thermonuclear target will be reflected or scattered back
into the laser amplifiers. There is some disagreement on
exactly how much reflection this might be in a properly

designed experiment, but even very small reflections can
have disasterous consequences. At least the first generation of lasers for fusion will operate with linear or weakly saturating amplifiers so that there will be a rather
large residual gain in the amplifier chain for the reflected pulse. The reflected pulse is also focused to a
smaller area as it propagates back through the chain (Fig.
1). If backward amplification is not suppressed, one can
guarantee that at some point in the chain the energy flux
in the reflected pulse will be high enough to damage optical components, a point which has been verified experimentally in a number of laboratories.

Amplifiers

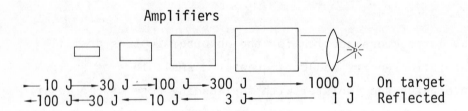

	On target
—10 J—→30 J—→100 J—→300 J——→ 1000 J	On target
—100 J—30 J——10 J—— 3 J———— 1 J	Reflected

Fig. 1. *The target reflection problem. Even a
very weak target reflection is amplified
and focused through the laser chain to
levels which exceed the design threshold
for components damage.*

Saturable absorbers with very fast recovery times
might be used to suppress backward amplification, but present absorbers are not suitable. The most straightforward
technique (and the least likely to degrade beam quality) is
to insert unidirectional elements, such as Faraday rotation isolators, between stages of the amplifier. At

1.06 μm this is easily accomplished. At 10.6 μm it is
rather more difficult and has net yet been done; Faraday
isolators have been made at 10.6 μm using rotation in
InSb,[13] but two-quantum absorption to the conduction band
will put an intensity flux limit of $\sim 10^5$ w/cm^2 on an InSb
isolator,[14] and this is lower than one would like. Note
that Faraday isolators are not suitable for interstage
isolation to reduce superfluorescence losses in a large
amplifier. The magnetic energy stored in a large aperture
isolator is large ($\sim$ 50 kj for a representative 30 cm
aperture isolator used for 1.06 μm at Lawrence Livermore
Laboratories) and cannot be switched in the nanosecond
times which interstage isolation requires.

There is an untested but promising technique for
eliminating the target reflection problem completely (Fig.
2). The high energy output pulse from the laser is first
passed through a nonlinear optical element, for example a
frequency doubler, and is then focused on the target.
Target reflections at 2ω pass back through the doubler
and arrive at the amplifier with components at 2ω and 4ω ,
but none within the amplifier gain bandwidth. There is
then no amplification of the reflected pulse. Conversion
efficiencies for doubling of $\sim$ 50% have been measured,
at very high intensities, so the insertion loss of such an
isolator is tolerable.

Wavelength Dependence Of Light Absorption
By An Imploding Thermonuclear Pellet

Absorption of intense light pulses by a dense hot
plasma is currently a very active field for theoretical
and experimental studies, and the various processes are

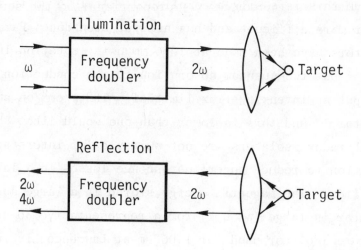

— Reflected beam can be separated by dispersive element
  or filter
— Will not be amplified by laser

Fig. 2. Target isolation by a nonlinear optical element.

not yet completely understood. The situation will become
much clearer when a body of experimental data from lasers
of higher intensity than those now operating become
available.

    For the present we can say that the most important
absorption processes--inverse bremsstrahlung and plasma
instabilities[15]--will deposit the laser energy in the low
density atmosphere blown off the surface of an imploding
pellet. Most of the energy deposition is at a point in
the atmosphere where the plasma frequency is near the laser frequency. Electrons are heated by the absorption and
electron thermal conduction carries energy to the core of
the imploding pellet.

The plasma frequency is proportional to the square root of the density so that low frequency radiation is absorbed far out in the atmosphere of the pellet rather than near the core. In some models[16] this could lead to decoupling of the atmosphere from the core and less transfer of energy to the high density regions where it is required. If true, this would suggest that short wavelengths are required to minimize the laser energy requirements for fusion. Other approximations[17] predict that electron thermal conduction through the intervening atmosphere to the core is sufficiently fast that the density at which the energy is deposited is not an important effect for laser wavelengths as long as 10.6 μm.

Instabilities in laser-heated plasmas may also contribute to decoupling of hot electrons from the pellet core. These instabilities are predicted to have a lower threshold for long wavelengths.[18]

In summary, theoretical studies indicate that short wavelengths are desirable for heating imploding pellets, but that 10.6 μm may not be too long a wavelength for the purpose.

Efficiency And Cost Of Operation

There are really two classes of laser fusion experiments which must concern us. Initial tests of fusion conditions can be done with any laser capable of producing the required pulse: net energy output and low cost are secondary considerations. If laser fusion is ever to be used as an economically competitive power source, however, the laser must convert energy efficiently and must have a low

operating cost. It is premature to discuss practical re-
actors, but current conceptual models of laser fusion re-
actors tend to imply a laser operating at about ten pulses/
sec and with an efficiency of at least a few percent.
Maintenance, such as the replacement of short-lived components, must also be inexpensive.

A pulse repetition rate of ten pulses/sec in a
large amplifier will be very difficult to achieve in any
laser other than a gas laser which can be cooled by convection, and a gas laser will probably be required for
such applications.

Summary: The "Ideal" Laser For Fusion

Figure 3 shows schematically the features which are
most desirable for a high energy storage, short-pulse laser, summarizing the previous discussion and adding a few
points which have been implied, but not specifically mentioned. In some laser systems the upper laser level will
be pumped directly.

The upper laser state should be pumped easily and
efficiently, implying a strong pumping transition which
couples well to the electrons or photons which supply the
pump energy. The upper laser level should have an inversion lifetime long enough for convenient pumping and high
energy storage.

Inversion lifetimes of $\sim 10^{-6}$ sec are probably
workable, but much shorter lifetimes are very difficult to
handle in a high energy device. Even longer inversion
lifetimes, in the hundreds of microseconds or milliseconds,
are very desirable.

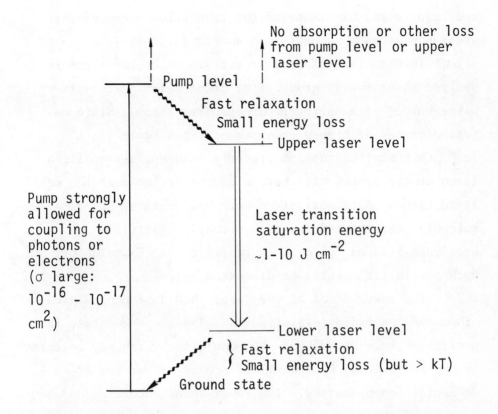

Fig. 3. The "ideal" high energy storage, high efficiency
         laser.

Energy storage at high energy density is desirable
to minimize the size of the laser structure: high energy
lasers will be large, even with high density storage, and
the distances and optical components involved could become
unworkably large for energy storage at very low densities.

The stimulated emission cross section should be
small, but large enough that the amplifier will saturate
at a flux within the limits of materials technology, which
at present means a few j/cm^2. The cross section σ is
proportional to $\dfrac{<\mu>^2}{\Delta\omega}$, where μ is the transition moment

and $\Delta\omega$ is the bandwidth of the transition. Hence, for small σ, μ must be small or $\Delta\omega$ large.

In the near infrared or visible, $\sigma \sim 10^{-20}$ cm^2 is desired which for an atomic line of normal bandwidth implies $\sim 10^{-4}$ of an electric dipole transition. Since matrix elements of higher order transitions scale as $\alpha^2 \sim 10^{-4}$, this implies that an electric quadrupole transition in an atomic system will have a cross section near the desired value. Alternatively a very broad state such as a molecular excimer complex or a strongly collision-broadened line may give an appropriate σ. Examples of both possibilities will be discussed later.

The lower level of the laser should be unpopulated, of course. A rapid relaxation to a lower energy state is desirable since it removes any population which may collect in the lower level by superfluorescence or various other de-excitation processes. The lower level should be an energy $>> kT$ above the ground state to avoid thermal population.

For efficient operation the energy loss in relaxation from the pump level to laser upper level and from laser lower level to the ground state must be small, and the pumping photons or electrons (or whatever) must be generated and transferred efficiently.

Having now defined what characteristics are desired in a laser for fusion, we shall examine the three existing laser transitions which presently seem to have the most promise for such applications.

7.3.   LASERS FOR FUSION - THREE CURRENT CANDIDATES

The first candidate is neodymium in glass[19] - 1.06 μm characterized by the following properties: (see Fig. 4)

Transition: field induced (F → I: an octupole in the free ion)

Pumping photon: 0.5 - 0.9 μm

Stimulated emission cross section: $\sim 3 \times 10^{-20}$ cm^2

Energy storage: $\sim$ 500 j/liter

Inversion lifetime: 300 μsec

Energy flux limit (self-focusing and surface damage): $\sim$ 1 - 2 j/cm^2 at present

Saturation energy flux (subnanosecond pulse): 6 j/cm^2)

Efficiency (for a practical subnanosecond amplifier): 0.2%

Average power: very low ($\sim$ 1 pulse every 15 min. in a large system)

Maximum output reported: $\sim$ 350 j 0.1 - 0.2 nsec (NRL, University of Rochester); $\sim$ 350 - 500 j 1 nsec (several labs)

Scalability (now under construction or in advanced design): $\sim 10^3$ j amplifier; $\sim 10^4$ j system

Discussion

Neodymium glass is the best current choice for laboratory feasibility studies of laser-plasma interactions and laser fusion. The technology of neodymium glass lasers is better developed than that for any competitive laser system, and a 10^3 - 10^4 joule 0.1 nsec system can be designed with high confidence. The 1.06 μm output of the laser may be easily converted to other frequencies (1.9 μm

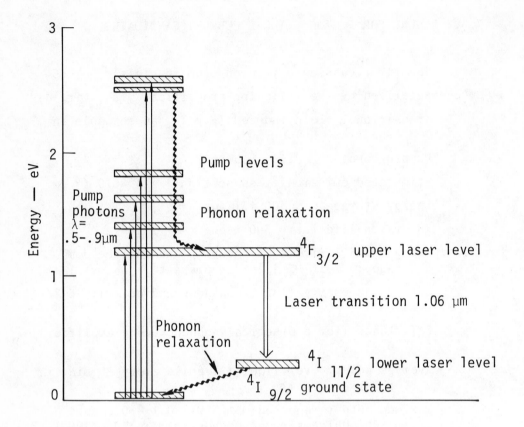

Fig. 4. Energy levels of the Nd^{3+} *in glass laser.*

by Raman scattering in H_2, 0.53 μm and 0.26 μm by frequency multiplication) with efficiencies of 20-50%, allowing
wavelength dependence studies of plasma interaction effects, optical component damage, and other areas which
must be well understood to determine what laser might be
suitable for a practical laser fusion device or for any
other applications of high energy subnanosecond pulses.

Neodymium glass will not be suitable for a practical laser fusion power plant or any other such application
which requires high efficiency, low cost per shot, and
high pulse rate. Cooling in glass is very slow, implying

a slow pulse rate. The efficiency in existing short pulse
neodymium lasers is also very poor. Present short pulse
lasers run at power densities $\sim$ 1 j/cm^2, which is much
less than the saturation flux: this avoids pulse distortion in a saturating amplifier (as well as two-photon absorption and self-focusing in the presently available
glasses), but further reduces the efficiency of the device.
The large stored energy remaining behind in the laser amplifiers also makes the target reflection problem more
severe since it increases the gain for the reflected pulse.

A neodymium laser requires that the optical beam
travel long distances through glass and other dense optical components for which nonlinearities in the index of
refraction are high. Self-focusing and the consequent
catastrophic damage to very expensive glass components is a
serious problem in these devices and sets very close tol-
erances on irregularities in the optics and in the pulse as
it propagates through the amplifiers.

A 1 - 0.1 nsec, 1 kj neodymium laser design[19] is
shown schematically in Fig. 5. A single 1 - 0.1 nsec
pulse is switched out of a mode-locked oscillator and amplified in a chain of solid rod amplifiers to an energy of
$\sim$ 10 j. A series of disc amplifiers, each with an energy
gain   3.5, amplifies the pulse to 1 kj. Each disc amplifier incorporates a polarizer and Faraday rotator to reduce coupling between stages and to suppress backward gain
which could amplify stray signals or target reflection
pulses. Such a 1 kj laser is presently under construction
at the Lawrence Livermore Laboratory, and an expansion to
10 kj using twelve parallel 1 kj chains of this type is
planned.

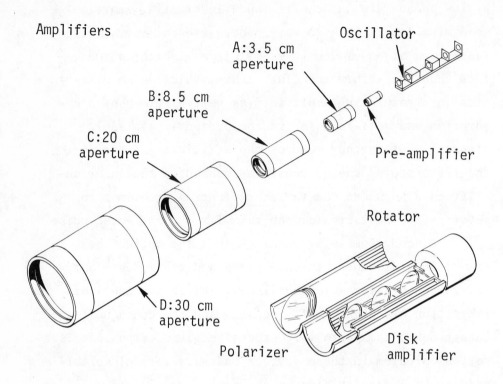

Fig. 5. *Schematic of 1 kj 100 picosecond neodymium laser chain.*

Other short-pulse, high energy neodymium lasers for laser fusion research are under development at the University of Rochester, Naval Research Laboratory, Compagnie Generale d'Electricite' (France), Lebedev Institute (USSR), KMS Fusion, Los Alamos Scientific Laboratory, and several other institutions.

The second candidate is the CO_2 - N_2 - He gas laser at 10.6 μm (see Fig. 6), characterized by the following properties:

Transition: vibrational intercombination

Pumping: electrons ($\sim$ 2 eV) $\rightarrow N_2^*$ $\rightarrow CO_2^*$; collisional relaxation of the lower level with He, N_2, CO_2.

| | Total Gas Pressure | |
	1 atm	3 atm
Stimulated emission cross section (for a single line)	1.5×10^{-18}cm^2	0.5×10^{-18}cm^2

Energy storage (CO_2 only):

multiline	$\sim$10 j/liter	$\sim$30 j/liter
single line	$\sim$0.7 j/liter	$\sim$2 j/liter

Inversion lifetime	20 µsec	7 µsec

Energy flux limit:

gas breakdown ($n_e \sim 10^{13}$)	$\sim$10 j/cm^2	$\sim$3 j/cm^2
optics	$\sim$3 j/cm^2	$\sim$3 j/cm^2

Saturation flux	0.013 j/cm^2	0.04 j/cm^2

(for each rotation-vibration
line: if energy is extracted
from more than one J state,
multiply by the number of
states).

Efficiency:

multiline, 1 µsec pulse: 3 - 5%

average power: high (flowing gas)

Maximum output reported: 150 j, 2 nsec (Los Alamos)
                         millijoules < 1 nsec

Scalability (now under construction or in design): 500 - 1000 j 1-2 nsec amplifier; $\sim 10^4$ j system

Discussion

The 10.6 µm carbon dioxide laser has an order of magnitude higher efficiency than any other current candidate for laser fusion. This alone makes it worth exploring. Optical components--modulators, isolators, saturable absorbers, etc.,--are not so well developed at 10.6 µm as they are at 1.06 µm, though the situation is improving.

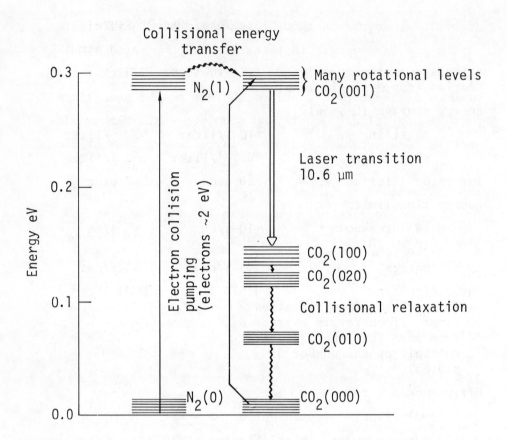

Fig. 6. *Energy levels of the* N_2 *-* CO_2 *- He gas laser.*

The 3 - 5% efficiency quoted may seem low to those who have heard figures nearer 20 - 30% for CO_2 lasers. For the nanosecond pulses of interest the only energy which can be extracted from the laser is that which is actually stored in the CO_2 first vibrational level: the energy stored in N_2 vibrations or in highly-excited CO_2 vibrations which could be extracted in microsecond pulses is lost here. For pulses $\leq \sim 2$ nsec an oscillation on a single rotation-vibration line of CO_2 will not be able to extract even all of the energy stored in the CO_2, since rotational relaxation to fill the upper level and empty the lower level occurs on about this time scale. Efficient extraction may require that the laser be operated simultaneously on a number of CO_2 lines. It is difficult to produce high energy CO_2 pulses shorter than 1 nsec since present optical components and modulators are rather slow and the lasers cannot support a large energy flux at the very high pressures needed to overlap the rotation-vibration lines.

The electron beam pulser-sustainer discharge in which the active medium is preionized by an electron beam and pumped by a high current, low voltage discharge seems to be the best choice for large CO_2 amplifiers. Smaller amplifier stages may use the simpler ultraviolet-preionized TEA laser discharges.

Los Alamos Scientific Laboratory is constructing a large CO_2 nanosecond pulse laser system, as discussed by Keith Boyer. Smaller scale efforts are underway at Lawrence Livermore Laboratory, Defense Research Establishment Valcartier (Canada) and other laboratories.

The third candidate is the iodine photodissociation laser at 1.315 μm (see Fig. 7), characterized by the following properties:

Transition: magnetic dipole, $I(^2P_{1/2}) \rightarrow I(^2P_{3/2})$, to the atomic ground state.

Pumping: photolysis (0.275 ± .05 μm) of CF_3I, C_2F_5I, and other iodides; absorption $\sigma \sim 5 \times 10^{-19}$ cm^2.

Optical cross section: at low pressure 2×10^{-18} cm^2; collision broadened in 1-3 atm He, 2×10^{-19} cm^2.

Energy storage: 25 j/liter.

Inversion lifetime: ~ 1000 μsec.

Damage limit (optics): 1 - 10 j/cm^2. (gas breakdown: ≥ 100 j/cm^2).

Saturation energy flux: 0.08 j/cm^2 at low pressure; 0.8 j/cm^2 in 1-3 atm He.

Efficiency (10 ns pulse: should be the same for shorter pulses): 0.5%.

Average power: high (flowing gas).

Maximum output (reported to date): $\sim$ 15 j, 10 nsec; 0, 0.1 nsec.

Scalability (defined to): 1 nsec 200 j amplifier, 1 nsec 1 kj system.

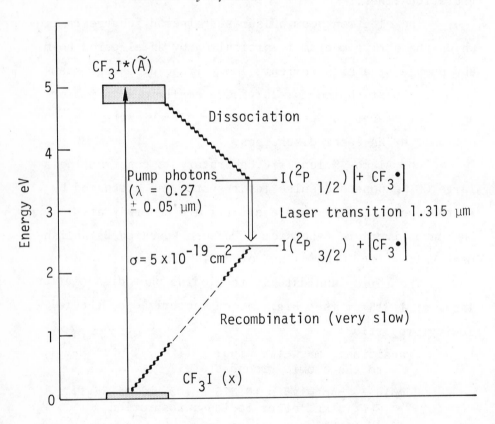

Fig. 7.   *Energy levels of the iodine photodissociation laser.*

Discussion

The iodine photodissociation laser is the least developed of the three systems considered here. So long as
the efficiency is comparable to neodymium glass it does
not seem too profitable to replace neodymium glass devices
with iodine for initial plasma interaction experiments,
particularly since the high gain of the iodine laser makes
engineering very difficult. The iodine line might be
broadened to lower the cross section even more by adding
10-20 atmospheres of helium or argon rather than one or
two atmospheres as has already been done, but three-body
reactions will begin to affect the kinetics in the laser
quite seriously at such high pressures, and these kinetics
are not well enough understood to predict the result un-
ambiguously without experimental confirmation.

The efficiency of the iodine laser might be raised
by an order of magnitude or so with careful matching of a
photolytic lamp to the $CF_3I(\tilde{A})$ continuum, and a high efficiency might make it worthwhile to design around the high
small signal gain of the iodine line. The photodissociation continuum of the alkyl iodides absorbs at most 8% of
the 10,000°K blackbody radiation from a xenon flashlamp
which converts $\sim$ 30-50% of the input electrical energy to
radiation, and this low transfer efficiency is responsible
for the low efficiency of the laser. The basic quantum
efficiency of iodine is a high 20%. A selective radiator
which radiates $\sim$ 50% of the input energy into the CF_3I,
C_2F_5I, C_3F_7I, etc., absorption continua could raise the
overall efficiency to $\sim$ 10%. The low cross section for
absorption into the $\tilde{A}$ continuum implies that a significant

amount of energy could still be lost to absorption in
other components of the laser, however. A possible photolytic lamp which couples very well to the $\tilde{A}$ continuum is
the (Hg-Xe) excimer (Hg^3P_o metastable-ground state Xe)
which radiates near 0.275 μm with a linewidth of 0.01 μm.
It is not known whether such radiation can be generated
efficiently.

One might attempt dissociation of CF_3I to yield
$I(^2P_{1/2})$ with electron collisions in a discharge, but this
technique will probably fail. The extra degrees of free-
dom which are available in an electron collision process
(i.e., the spin, angular momentum, and energy of the electron leaving the collision) makes such collisions less
selective than photolysis. Any loss of selectivity will
cause a yield of $I(^2P_{3/2})$ which is not only subtracted
from the upper level population but. is added to the laser
lower level, and is therefore doubly damaging. Spin exchange between fine structure levels such as $I(^2P_{3/2})$ and
$I(^2P_{1/2})$ is also very fast in collisions with low energy
electrons. Spin relaxation among the fine structure
states of the neon $2p^53s$ configuration,[57] for example, has
a cross section near $10^{-14}cm^2$. Chemical population of the
$^2P_{3/2}$ state has been proposed to explain some experimental
observations of gain in iodine lasers,[21] but diffusion of
excited atoms in the active medium can easily explain
these observations.[23] The efficiency of an iodine laser
for practical applications must of course include the energy cost of manufacture and purification of the CF_3I or
other iodine source. Even if the active molecules are re-
formed by recombination of the radicals (which has been
detected) some purification will be required, and the

system is sensitive to small concentrations of contaminants such as molecular iodine or oxygen.

At the present time the chief center of iodine laser development is the Max Planck Institut für Plasma-Physik (Garching, Germany) where the 15 j, 10 nsec amplifier discussed above was constructed. A 1 kj system consisting of six parallel 200 j amplifiers is now under construction.

7.4. EXCIMER LASERS

General Discussion

There is a large class of excimer molecular systems in which some electronically excited molecular states formed by one atom in its ground state and a second atom in an electronically excited state are bound but the molecular ground state is not, as shown schematically in Fig. 8. A population inversion is established automatically in these systems when an excited state is populated. The molecule in its ground state flies apart on a dissociative curve in a time comparable to one vibrational period ($\sim 10^{-12}$ sec) so excimer molecules represent one of the very few systems in which relaxation effects can influence energy extraction in a 10^{-10} sec pulse. The practical advantage of the dissociation is that a photon can be extracted from each excited molecule which is formed rather than only enough photons to equalize the population in the upper and lower levels.

The lower level of the excimer must, however, be empty in fact rather than in principle. As shown in Fig.

8b, some excimer ground states have a structure which allows molecules colliding at thermal energies to ride up the
repulsive curve to an internuclear separation which puts
them into the region for vertical transitions to the bound
excited state. These collision complexes then absorb the
photons emitted by the excimer and represent, in effect, a
ground state population which reduces the population
inversion.

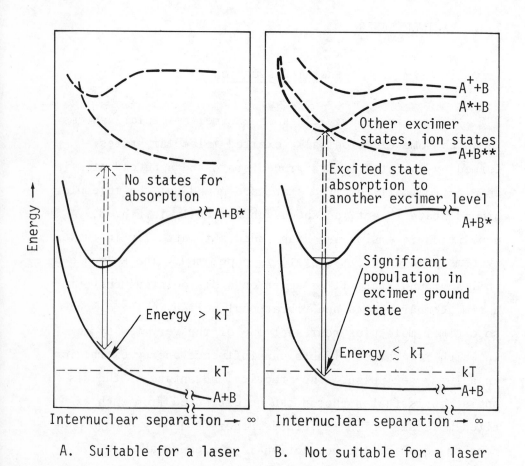

Fig. 8. Typical excimer energy levels.

Many excimers also have bound levels, or a photoionization or photodissociation continuum, at an energy
which can be reached by absorption of a laser photon from
the upper level of the laser transition. The effect of
this excited state absorption depends on the relative cross
sections for absorption of this state and stimulated emission down to the ground state, but it is obviously an un-
desirable feature. The visible excimer continuum in mer-
cury vapor may suffer from this problem[24] and the rare gas
excimer lasers almost surely do, though obviously it does
not prevent laser oscillation in these systems.

The emission from an excimer bound-repulsive transition is typically a very broad continuum. The integrated
line strength may be quite high, but the large bandwidth
implies that the optical cross section and hence the small-
signal gain is low in any small frequency interval. This
of course makes demonstration of laser oscillation somewhat
more difficult, but, as we have discussed, it is desirable
for a large amplifier.

Excimer radiation can also be very efficiently generated under some circumstances. Measurements of the rare
gas excimer radiation at a low density of excitation indicate that $\sim$ 30-50% of the energy deposited in a rare gas by
a high energy charged particle can be converted to excimer
fluorescence under the proper circumstances. Rare gas
excimer lasers to date have been operated at rather high
excimer densities and have shown correspondingly lower
efficiencies, on the order of 1%. Note, however, that even
this efficiency is not exceptionally low when compared to
other available short wavelength lasers. The loss of efficiency at high densities of excitation comes from excimer

collision processes such as

$$Xe_2^* + Xe_2^* \rightarrow Xe_2^+ + Xe + Xe + e$$

which deplete the energy stored in the Xe_2^* excimers before it can be extracted by the laser pulse.

Rare Gas Excimer Lasers

Laser oscillation has been demonstrated on the excimer continua of pure Xe_2^* and Kr_2^* excited by electron
beam radiolysis,[26] and on the excimer continuum of xenon in
a radiolysed mixture of Ar and Xe in which xenon is the
minority constituent. In the latter case the energy
transfer

$$Ar_2^* + Xe \rightarrow Ar + Ar + Xe^*$$

$$M + Xe^* + Xe \rightarrow M + Xe_2^*$$

transfers energy very efficiently to the xenon excimer,
while the effect of xenon excimer ground state absorption
is much reduced. (Fig. 9)

Impurities can be a very serious problem in rare gas
excimer lasers. Note, for example, that xenon has two resonance lines, one of which lies at 1470 Å in the Kr_2^* continuum and one at 1236 Å in the Ar_2^* continuum. Xenon is
always present in commercial samples of these gases at the
level of a few parts per million, and its presence at that

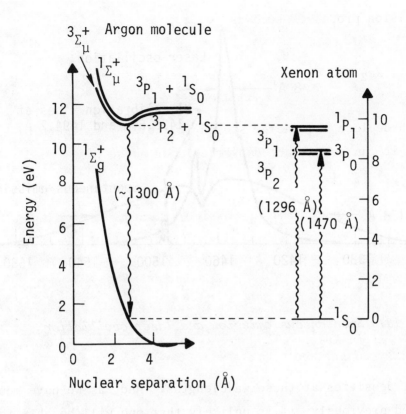

Fig. 9. Resonant transfer $Ar_2^* \rightarrow Xe$ ($^1P_1$).

level can substantially influence the laser oscillation and
energy transfer kinetics of these mixtures. Figure 10
shows for example the Kr_2^* continuum below and above laser
oscillation threshold as seen in the authors' laboratory
with a prominent absorption feature from the 1470 Å resonance line of a minute xenon impurity. One is also often
able to detect absorptive features from such species as CO.

It is very difficult to obtain high quality mirrors
in the vacuum ultraviolet, and severe mirror damage with
evaporation of the MgF_2 substrate and aluminum reflector is
common in these lasers. Very careful surface finishing is
required to fabricate mirrors which will withstand high

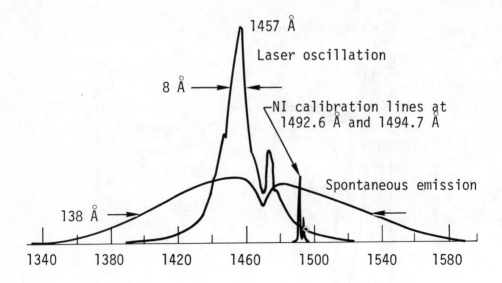

Fig. 10. Spontaneous emission and laser oscillation in Kr_2^*.

power densities at these wavelengths. And, as we have mentioned previously, it is unlikely that one will be able to transmit a high energy flux at wavelengths this short through reasonable optical elements. The rare gas excimers are the best understood of the excimer systems, however, and a study of them can test the importance of various kinetic processes and give information useful for other potential excimer lasers.

We shall not discuss the experimental results on rare gas excimer lasers in any detail here. For further information one may consult the papers listed in Ref. 26.

Other Potential Excimer Lasers

A few of the many known excimer emission continua are listed in Table 2. Some of these may be suitable for laser oscillation if they avoid the problems discussed above and if the kinetics of an active medium can be arranged to generate them efficiently.

TABLE 2

REPRESENTATIVE GAS-PHASE EXCIMER CONTINUA

Species	Peak λ	Comments	Reference
Xe_2^*	1720	Laser	(26) (27)
Kr_2^*	1457	Laser	(26) (27)
Ar_2^*	1300		(27)
Hg_2^*	3350		(28)
Hg_2^*	4850	Excited State Absorption	(24) (28)
$HgXe^*$	2750		(22)
$Hg(H_2O)^*$	2900		(22)
$Hg(NH_3)^*$	3500		(22)
ArH^*	7670 ⎱	Bound, Predisso-	(29) (30)
XeO^*	5450 ⎰	ciated Lower State	
HeH, NeH, etc. ⎱			
$LiHe$, $LiXe$, etc. ⎬		Predicted, but not yet observed	(31)
$NaHe$, $NaXe$, etc. ⎰			

The spectra of excimer molecules are very complex and there are many opportunitites for error in the identification of excimer states and even excimer species. It has been noted,[32] for example, that some spectral features which have at times been identified with the Hg_2^* excimer are probably due to HgCl and CN. Some of the visible continua observed in, for example, xenon discharges[33] are probably from the XeO excimer, or the unidentified but presumably quite similar XeC and XeN excimers, rather than from levels in a pure xenon excimer species. Impurities of any of these atoms are usually found even in very clean vacuum systems.

Energy Transfer From Excimers

The broad bandwidth of excimer transitions allows resonant energy transfer to a wide variety of other species in a gas. An example of such transfer as shown in Fig. 10 is the argon excimer to xenon atom transfer already mentioned, a process which has a cross section[26] near 10^{-13} cm^2. Even those excimers which are not suitable for a high energy storage laser may be useful in a kinetic chain for populating a specific level in some other laser device, either by collision transfer or by photolytic decomposition with the efficient excimer fluorescence. We have mentioned a possible application of the $(Hg\ Xe)^*$ excimer to the iodine photodissociation laser in this regard and will discuss another example in the next section.

7.5. A POSSIBLE LASER ON THE AURORAL LINE OF OXYGEN

General Discussion Of Candidate Atoms
For A High Energy Storage Atomic Laser

We have indicated that a laser for fusion research
should ideally be a gas laser with a short wavelength and
at least a few μsec energy storage time, should be free of
excited state absorption and other losses from the upper
laser level, and should have a stimulated emission cross
section near that which is predicted for an electric quadrupole electronic transition. In addition one wishes a
potential for reasonably high efficiency of at least a few
percent. An atomic system has an advantage for picosecond
pulses, since all the energy is stored in a single state
and can be extracted without requiring relaxation process
to occur. In an atomic system these conditions imply that
one wants a low lying "metastable" level as an upper laser
state, no atomic levels above this level up to energies so
high that absorption from the upper laser level or collision of two metastable atoms cannot depopulate the upper
level, and an efficient source of the appropriate metastable level, all of which are implied in Fig. 3.

A quick analysis of atomic spectra suggests that
these conditions are fulfilled in atoms with a partially
filled P shell in which the Pauli Principle prevents an
arrangement of electrons in the lowest electron configuration to give allowed electric dipole transitions among the
electronic levels of this configuration, but in which the
energy required to promote an electron to the next S shell
is so large that the effect of higher excited states in the

atom can be ignored. These conditions prevail in the
fourth, fifth, and sixth columns of the periodic table, or
in the first period in carbon, oxygen, and nitrogen.

The Oxygen Atom

Figure 11 shows the three electronic levels of the
$2p^4$ electron configuration of oxygen, which is the best
studied of these potential laser species and the one which
at first glance looks most promising,[34] though others may
also prove suitable. Both the $^1S_0$ and the $^1D_2$ state are
radiatively metastable in the dipole approximation, but all
of the possible "forbidden" higher order lines have been
detected and are labeled in the figure. These lines are
important in atmospheric and astrophysical phenomena which
has led to the common names shown. The electric quadrupole "auroral" green line is in fact the most prominent
visible atomic line in the night sky emission from the atmosphere and the largest contributor to the luminosity of
most auroral displays.[35]

Table 3 shows the rate of reaction or deactivation
of the $^1S_0$ and $^1D_2$ states with various molecules, giving a
measure of the ability of these states to survive collisions in a gas.[36] Note that the $^1S_0$ state is highly re-
sistant to deactivation in collisions with a wide variety
of gas molecules and that the $^1D_2$ state is much less stable. As an example, if excited oxygen atoms are produced
in otherwise pure molecular nitrogen at one atmosphere
pressure, the $1/e$ decay time for the $^1S_0$ state will be
longer than $\sim$ 800 μsec while for the $^1D_2$ state the decay
time will be some five orders of magnitude less or $\sim$ 2 nsec.

One may, therefore, maintain an inverted population on the auroral transition for some microseconds in nitrogen or in a variety of other gases if the concentration of rapidly reacting molecules such as H_2O or NO is carefully controlled.

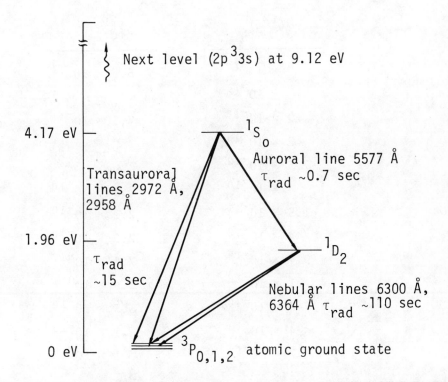

Next level ($2p^3 3s$) at 9.12 eV

4.17 eV

$^1S_0$

Auroral line 5577 Å
τ_{rad} ~0.7 sec

Transauroral lines 2972 Å, 2958 Å

1.96 eV

$^1D_2$

τ_{rad} ~15 sec

Nebular lines 6300 Å, 6364 Å τ_{rad} ~110 sec

0 eV

$^3P_{0,1,2}$ atomic ground state

Fig. 11. *Energy levels of the lowest electron configuration in atomic oxygen ($2p^4$).*

Another important collision property of an excited atom is its rate of reaction on collision with a second excited atom, since this rate sets an upper bound on the density of excited atoms which can be maintained. For the collision between $^1S_0$ oxygen atoms there are in principle two channels available for deactivation, the excitation transfer

TABLE 3

DEACTIVATION OF THE METASTABLE SINGLET STATES OF OXYGEN

Rate Constants[36] for $\sim$ 300°K in units of cm^3 molecule^{-1}sec^{-1}

	$O(^1S_0)$	$O(^1D_2)$
N_2	$< 5 \times 10^{-17}$	5.5×10^{-11}
$N(^4S)$	$\leq 10^{-12}$	--
O_2	2×10^{-13}	7.5×10^{-11}
$O(3p)$	2×10^{-13}; 7.5×10^{-12}	--
NO	4×10^{-10}	2.1×10^{-10}
N_2O	1.5×10^{-11}	2.2×10^{-10}
CO_2	4×10^{-13}	2.2×10^{-10}
CO	9.4×10^{-14}	7.5×10^{-11}
H_2	1×10^{-15}	2.9×10^{-11}
H_2O	4×10^{-10}	3.5×10^{-10}
He	$< 4 \times 10^{-19}$	$\sim 1 \times 10^{-15}$
Xe	6.7×10^{-15}	$\sim 1 \times 10^{-10}$

$$O(^1S) + O(^1S) \to O^* \text{ (higher states)} + O(^3P, {}^1D)$$

and molecular formation

$$O(^1S) + O(^1S) \to O_2^+ + e,$$

$$M + O(^1S) + O(^1S) \to O_2 + M.$$

The available energy for two colliding ^1S_O atoms is 8.34 eV, while the nearest higher excited state of the oxygen is at 9.12 eV, giving an energy defect of some .78 eV for excitation transfer. This argues that the excitation transfer rate will be negligible at any reasonable gas temperature. Theoretical treatments of molecular formation in a collision between two $O(^1S_O)$ atoms indicate that this is also a very unlikely process. Two $O(^1S_O)$ atoms collide on a repulsive surface which does not cross any lower energy bound state surface of the oxygen molecule or ion at energies up to $\sim$ 3 eV, which is far above thermal energies. There are no quantitative data available to confirm these predictions, but it appears from the information presently available that upper-laser-level excited-state collisions will have a negligible influence on the kinetics of an auroral line laser, unlike, for example, the Xe_2^* excimer laser.

The stimulated emission cross section for the auroral transition is evaluated from the usual expression for line strength given in Sec. 7.2 and for a doppler-broadened line at 300°K is 9×10^{-20} cm^2 at line center.

The saturation energy $\frac{h\nu}{\sigma}$ is $\sim$ 4 j/cm^2, ignoring the effects of level degeneracy in the $^1D_2$ level, which may be expected to influence the saturation behavior.

Oxygen Excimers

Oxygen in the ^1S and ^1D states forms excimer molecules with the rare gases, N_2, and probably other molecules. Analysis of excimer band spectra of XeO indicates[30] that the state correlating to $O(^1S_O)$ is weakly bound (~ 0.06 eV for XeO), while the $O(^1D_2)$ state is more tightly bound (~ 0.34 eV). The state correlating to $O(^3P)$ is repulsive and crosses the $O(^1D_2)$ state, leading to rapid nonradiative decay. Laser oscillation has been seen in a similar situation[37] in NO. At first glance the states do not look promising for laser oscillation in XeO or similar excimers, however. The kinetic data for deactivation of $O(^1S)$ (by, for example, Xe or N_2) suggest a slow rate of formation combined with a fast radiative lifetime, so that it is difficult to generate a high density of the excited excimer species.

Note that oxygen excimer radiation is blue-shifted since the $[Xe - O(^1D_2)]$ complex is more tightly bound than $[Xe - O(^1S_O)]$.

Populating The ^1S State of Oxygen: Kr_2^* - N_2O Transfer

Many reactions are known to produce $O(^1S_O)$, but the yields and efficiencies are not all quantitatively understood. We shall present one example of a potential laser medium here; many others are possible but are not so well characterized.

The N_2O molecule has a photodissociative continuum[38] at 1450 Å with a half intensity width of some 75 Å and a peak absorption cross section of 6×10^{-18} cm^2. Photolytic yields[39] at 1470 Å within this continuum are shown in Table 4. There is a high efficiency for production of $O(^1S)$ plus a yield of several other products, the yields for which are not so well known since they are more difficult to detect than $O(^1S)$. The Kr_2^* excimer fluoresces

TABLE 4

YIELD[39] FROM PHOTOLYSIS OF N_2O AT 1470 Å

$N_2O + h\nu \rightarrow$	yield
$N_2(x) + O(^1S)$	0.5 ± 0.1
$N_2(x) + O(^1D)$	≤ 0.55
$NO(x) + N(^2D)$	$0.02 \pm 0.02; \geq 0.0003$
$N_2(A) + O(^3P)$	0.08 ± 0.02
TOTAL	1.00

Note: This table assumes that spin conservation is strictly obeyed. If it is not, $O(^3P)$ and $N(^2D)$ yields may change.

efficiently in a continuum centered at 1460 Å which couples very well to this N_2O absorption with an effective cross section of $\sim 3 \times 10^{-18}$ cm^2.

Photolysis of N_2O with Kr_2^* radiation in the presence of a background concentration of N_2 or rare gases to collisionally quench $O(^1D)$ and thermalize hot atoms appears, therefore, to be a reasonable candidate for an auroral line laser. From Tables 3 and 4 one may predict an inversion lifetime ~ 8 μsec for $O(^1S)$ produced by photolysis of $\sim 10^{16}$ cm^{-3} concentration of N_2O in a background of one atmosphere of nitrogen. The energy storage in such a system will be about one j/liter. Neither the inversion lifetime nor the energy storage is as high as one might like, but also neither one is unreasonable. Many deactivation processes[40] have an activation energy large enough to give a strong temperature dependence, and deactivation by these species can be reduced by chilling the active medium. Unfortunately the chief offender in this system, NO, reacts with no apparent activation energy.

A Kr_2^* - N_2O collision will also produce $O(^1S)$ with yields which may not be too different from those of Table 4. There will be some loss of selectivity since there are many more channels available for the products of a collision than for a photolytic process in which the energy, spin states, and the like are well defined.

Other Sources Of $O(^1S)$

Photolysis of CO_2 near 1150 Å has a yield[41] of $O(^1S)$ which is $(75 \pm 25)\%$ and is thought to be 100%. There are problems here, however: no efficient, fast source of 1150 Å radiation has been identified and it is rather unlikely that the very high flux from a photolytic lamp intense enough to drive a high energy storage amplifier can be passed through a window at this wavelength. Collision transfer processes in a discharge containing CO_2 may be suitable for producing $O(^1S)$: some $O(^1S)$ has been detected in collisional dissociation of CO_2 by argon metastables,[42] though the principal product of such transfer appears to be $CO(a^3\pi) + O(^3P)$. The subsequent collisional energy transfer of $CO(a^3\pi)$ colliding with $O(^3P)$ has a very fast rate $(2 \times 10^{-10}$ cm^3/sec)[43] and theoretically has a high yield of $O(^1S)$,[44] so that $CO(a^3\pi)$ production may also be an efficient source of $O(^1S)$. No experimental data on the yield of $O(^1S)$ is available.

$O(^1S)$ is produced in large quantity in "active nitrogen" discharges with a small oxygen impurity.[45] The principal production mechanism, at low excitation density in a radiolytic discharge, has been shown to be an ionic reaction of very low activation energy.[46] Though the identity of the reaction is not certain, the evidence may favor $N^+ + O_2 \rightarrow NO^+ + O(^1S)$.

Towards An Auroral Line Laser

For the moment there is enough information available on the properties and excitation of $O(^1S)$ to make an auroral line laser look interesting, but not enough to determine whether such a laser will have high enough energy storage and efficiency to be practical. Such parameters as the collision broadening of the auroral line and the structure of oxygen excimers, photolytic yields as a function of wavelength within the N_2O photodissociative continuum (there is qualitative evidence that they vary) and reaction rates in an appropriate laser mixture under high intensity photolysis or intense discharge conditions must be determined to answer these questions.

7.6. TWO QUANTUM AMPLIFIERS

General Properties

We shall close these notes with a short discussion of a somewhat speculative laser device, the two-quantum amplifier. The single photon lasers which we have been discussing all suffer from superfluorescence and parasitic oscillation because of the presence of a large small signal gain for fluorescence in the amplifier. If an amplifier were designed to have gain only in the presence of an intense pulse of radiation, these limits to the size and energy storage density of a laser amplifier would be eliminated.

Figure 12 shows three variations on two-quantum systems which satisfy these conditions. In each case levels 1 and 2 are of the same parity so that the transition from 1 to 2 is dipole-forbidden and of such low amplitude that it may be neglected, and a population inversion is established between the upper level 1 and the lower level 2.

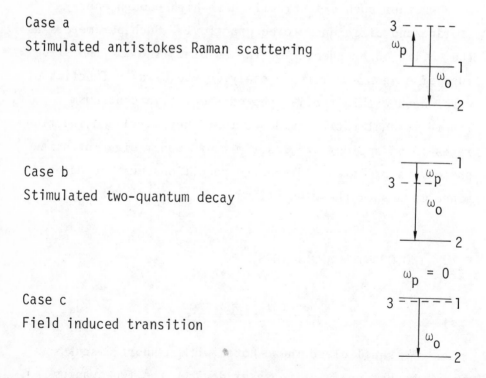

Case a
Stimulated antistokes Raman scattering

Case b
Stimulated two-quantum decay

Case c
Field induced transition

Fig. 12. *Potential two-quantum amplifiers.*

In case $\underline{a}$ we have stimulated antistokes Raman scattering[47] of a pump photon with emission of an antistokes photon at ω_o. Since one photon is absorbed at ω_p for each photon emitted at ω_o, the energy gain in a single stage is limited to $\frac{\omega_o}{\omega_p}$. If the process were allowed to proceed as an ordinary superfluorescent stimulated Raman amplifier, the intensity at ω_o would grow to the point that a second Raman scattering step would be possible, shifting ω_o to still higher frequencies, and the output would be multi-frequency and rather difficult to control. To avoid such effects a Raman upconversion amplifier will probably operate with input signals at both ω_p and ω_o and with an intensity flux at both of these frequencies which is below the threshold for superfluorescent scattering. Stimulated antistokes scattering is of course very common, but it has not yet been studied in a system inverted by some external agency rather than by a preexisting stimulated stokes scattering process.

Case $\underline{b}$ represents a two-quantum stimulated decay. The most interesting case would be for $\omega_o = \omega_p$ so that only a single strong field is required to drive the amplifier. Antistokes Raman scattering as in case $\underline{a}$ may have a higher cross section than two-quantum decay since the virtual intermediate state 3 may be nearer a real state of the system for the case of Raman scattering, so that Raman scattering may have to be carefully suppressed. A two-quantum transition such as this has been demonstrated for a resonant four-wave interaction in potassium vapor,[48] but not with significant amounts of energy storage.

Case $\underline{c}$ is antistokes Raman scattering in which the frequency of the pump photon is reduced to zero; that is,

it becomes a dc electric or magnetic field.[49] Both have
been demonstrated[50,51] (in non-inverted systems, however).
In solids, rather than the more interesting gases, these
transitions are common: the noedymium glass laser, for
example, is an induced transition.

Each of these three processes proceeds through an
intermediate virtual state 3 of opposite parity to 1 and 2,
and the amplitude for each process is enhanced if a real
state is present near the virtual state so that the energy
denominator is reduced in the perturbation expansion for
the amplitudes of the interaction. Resonant Raman scattering,[52] or the magnetic field-induced transition in mer-
cury[51] are examples in which a nearby state greatly en-
hances the cross section for the effect.

Demonstration In Atomic Iodine

Calculations[53] indicate that the stimulated Raman
gain on the iodine $^2P_{1/2}$ - $^2P_{3/2}$ transition used in the
iodine photodissociation laser is large. The equivalent
stimulated emission cross section for stimulated Raman
gain[49] is commonly expressed

$$\sigma(\nu) = \frac{4}{\pi} \frac{\lambda_s^2}{h\nu_\rho} I\rho \frac{\delta\sigma}{\delta\Omega} g(\nu)$$

where λ_s is the wavelength of the scattered radiation,
$h\nu_\rho$ and I_ρ are the photon energy and intensity of the
pump, $\frac{\delta\sigma}{\delta\Omega}$ is the differential Raman-scattering cross section, and $g(\nu)$ is the lineshape of the transition. The
differential cross section $\frac{\delta\sigma}{\delta\Omega}$ at the peak of the doppler

broadened iodine fine-structure line is predicted to be
$\sim 3.5 \times 10^{-28}$ cm^2/steradian for excitation at the 0.6943 μm
Ruby wavelength. A typical vibrational Raman scattering
cross section in hydrogen gas, for example, is only $\sim 10^{-29}$
cm^2 for excitation at this wavelength.

The 3.5×10^{-28} cm^2 cross section gives a gain of
some 15 cm^{-1} with a laser pump at 10^9 w/cm^2, assuming
steady-state scattering. The iodine transition is narrow,
however, and steady-state conditions do not apply for a
picosecond pulse. Transient scattering effects will lower
the gain by perhaps an order of magnitude.[54]

Several laboratories are investigating a possible
demonstration of stimulated Raman upconversion in iodine.
The system is probably not suitable for a practical amplifier since the ordinary single-quantum gain is so high that
even a laboratory demonstration Raman amplifier suffers
from severe superfluorescence and parasitics. Such an amplifier could be useful to test models of the nonlinear
optics of two-quantum transitions, however, and is being
pursued for that goal.[56]

Some Other Possibilities

Several other two-quantum amplifiers have been proposed, but as of now there are no proposals which have a
clear potential for development as practical high-energy
amplifiers. Two possibilities are mentioned below as they
illustrate some of the problems to be faced as well as some
desirable features for any future proposal for these
amplifiers.

We discussed earlier the very efficient excitation
of atomic xenon by argon excimer collision transfer. The
kinetics of the process may allow an inversion of the xenon $^3P_2$ metastable level with respect to the atomic ground
state. The $^3P_1$ upper level of the 0.1470 μm resonance
transition lies 977.6 cm^{-1} above the $^3P_2$ level, which is a
defect of $\sim$ 0.4 cm^{-1} for resonant Raman scattering of the
R(22) line of the 10.6 μm CO_2 laser (Fig. 9). The $^3P_0$ -
$^3P_1$ transition is a magnetic dipole, so the resonance enhancement is not so high as it would be for an electric
dipole resonant process, but it may allow the effect to be
observed. As we have discussed previously, however, the
resulting 0.146 μm wavelength is too short for a practical
high energy laser.

Vibrations in hydrogen, or other homonuclear molecules such as nitrogen, are efficiently excited by electron
collision and might prove useful for a stimulated Raman
amplifier. Figure 13 shows the appropriate states in parahydrogen. It is not possible to invert the Q branch transitions with a simple electron pumping scheme at any reasonable energy, since the population distribution simply
comes to the same temperature as the electron distribution.
The rotational temperature can stay low, however, so lines
such as the $0_1(2)$ are inverted. Such partial inversions
are common in, e.g., carbon monoxide lasers. Q branch
transitions in hydrogen might be inverted by anharmonic
V-V pumping (again, as seen in CO), but if conditions are
arranged to favor this pumping, the energy will be widely
distributed in the vibrational levels and will not be
available for short-pulse extraction in a single
transition.

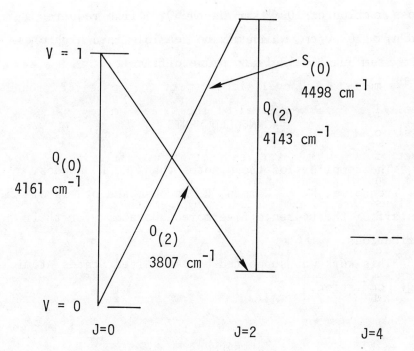

Fig. 13.   *Rotation-vibration energy levels of parahydrogen.*

If the Q lines are not inverted, a new parasitic oscillation problem arises to replace the superfluores-cence which we have eliminated.   The cross section for nor-mal Stokes stimulated Raman scattering on the Q(0) line is about a factor of three higher than the cross section for antistokes scattering on the 0(2) line.[55]   The amplifier must then be driven with two strong waves at the pump and at the scattered frequency and the amplitude for each of these waves must be low enough to avoid superfluorescent Raman oscillation on the Q(0) line (or on rotational tran-sitions).   We see therefore that a two-quantum amplifier does not necessarily eliminate parasitics.

Field-induced transitions corresponding to case 3 of Fig. 12 have been measured among these hydrogen levels.[50]

A cross section of 10^{-20} cm^2 on the O(2) line requires a field of $\sim 10^6$ v/cm, which may be feasible in a high pressure system but is likely to prove difficult.

ACKNOWLEDGMENTS

The compilers of these notes thank C. K. Rhodes, J. B. Trenholme, R. L. Carman, R. Jacobs, and others of the staff of the Lawrence Livermore Laboratory for their contributions.

This work was supported by the United States Atomic Energy Commission.

REFERENCES

1. See also J. Nuckolls, J. L. Emmett, and L. Wood, *Physics Today*, 26, 8, 46 (August 1973).

2. A. J. Glass and A. H. Guenther, *Appl. Opt.* 12, 637 (1973) and other papers in that Journal issue; also A. J. Glass and A. H. Guenther, Lawrence Livermore Laboratory Report UCRL-74813 (1973).

3. Self-focusing is discussed in more detail by S. A. Akhmanov, R. V. Khokhlov, and A. P. Sukhorukov, Chapter E3 of *Laser Handbook*, ed. by F. T. Arecchi and E. O. Schulz-Dubois, North Holland, Amsterdam (1972). See also M. M. T. Loy and Y. R. Shen, *IEEE J. Quant. Elect.* 9, 409 (1973); J. H. Marburger and E. L. Dawes, *Phys. Rev. Lett.* 21, 55 (1968); E. S. Bliss, *IEEE J. Quant. Elect.* QE8, 273 (1972) and in Ref. 2.

4. M. Bass and H. H. Barrett, *Appl. Opt.* 12, 690 (1973).

5. Private communications, C. Phipps, Y. L. Pan (LLL); W. Reichert (Los Alamos).

6. We use Eq. (7) of R. Braunstein and N. Ockman, *Phys. Rev.* 134, A499 (1964) thus assuming an "allowed-allowed", resonant absorption. Experimental results for 1.06 µm absorption tend to fall nearer the values predicted in this way than the values for less allowed processes.

7. A. Penzkofer and W. Kaiser, *Appl. Phys. Lett.* 21, 427 (1972).

8. Self-focusing at 50 atm in CO_2 and N_2O is described by M. E. Mack, et al., *Appl. Phys. Lett.* 16, 209 (1970). If the laser frequency is very near a resonance of the medium (such as if the lasing species is present in very high concentration), self-focusing may be more important. See A. Javan and P. L. Kelley, *IEEE J. Quant. Elect.* 2, 470 (1966). N. Karlov, et al., *JETP Letters* 17, 239 (1973) describe another resonant self-focusing phenomenon which may be too slow to influence subnanosecond pulses. See also J. E. Bjorkholm and A. Ashkin, *Phys. Rev. Letter* 32, 129 (1973).

9. Some recent experimental measurements are given by R. T. Brown and D. C. Smith, *Appl. Phys. Lett.* 22, 245 (1973) and P. J. Berger and D. C. Smith, *Appl. Phys. Lett.* 21, 167 (1972). S. D. Rockwood, G. H. Canavan, and W. A. Proctor, *IEEE J. Quant. Elect.* 9, 154 (1973) predict that the threshold may be less than these long pulse experimental values for subnanosecond pulses. E. Yablanovitch, *Appl. Phys. Lett.* 23, 121 (1973), connects these thresholds to DC breakdown parameters. The theory is treated by N. Kroll and K. Watson, *Phys. Rev.* A8, 804 (1973) and the references listed there.

10. Y. L. Pan, J. R. Simpson, and A. F. Bernhart, Lawrence Livermore Laboratory preprint UCRL 75078 (1973); submitted to *Appl. Phys. Lett.*

11. Pulse propagation in a saturating amplifier is discussed by L. M. Frantz and J. S. Nodvik, *J. Appl. Phys.* 34, 2346 (1973) for the case of a pulse long compared to the phase relaxation time of the amplifier. A more detailed treatment of this case is found in "A Simple Approach to Laser Amplifiers," J. B. Trenholme and K. R. Manes, Lawrence Livermore Laboratory Report UCRL 51413 (1972), available from *NTIS*. Pulse propagation for pulses short compared to the phase relaxation time is discussed by A. Icsevgi and W. E. Lamb, Jr., *Phys. Rev.* 185, 517 (1969). See also the chapters by F. Hopf and M. Sargent in this volume.

12. This rule-of-thumb represents, for example, the gain required to go above threshold for a diffuse parasitic in a cube-shaped amplifier with two open ends, assuming four 1% diffusely reflecting walls. See A. N. Chester, *Appl. Opt.* 12, 2139 (1973).

13. A. L. Mikaelyan, et. al., *Sov. J. Quant. Elect.* 1, 271 (1971).

14. J. M. Doviak, et al., *J. Phys.* C6, 593 (1973).

15. P. Kaw and J. Dawson, *Phys. Fluids* 12, 2586 (1969); W. Kruer and J. Dawson, *Phys. Fluids* 15, 446 (1972).

16. R. Kidder and J. Pink, *Nucl. Fusion* 12, 325 (1972).

17. See the chapter by R. Morse in this volume.

18. J. Katz, et al., Lawrence Livermore Laboratory Report UCRL 74334 (1972), J. Nuckolls, UCRL 74345 (1972), J. W. Shearer and J. J. Duderstadt UCRL 73717 (1972).

19. Factors influencing the design of short pulse neo-
    dymium amplifiers are discussed in detail in the fol-
    lowing: P. G. Kriukov and V. S. Letokhov, Chap. C3
    of *Laser Handbook*, ed. by F. T. Arecchi and E. O.
    Schulz-Dubois, North-Holland, Amsterdam (1972); J. M.
    McMahon, J. L. Emmett, J. F. Holzrichter, and J. B.
    Trenholme, *IEEE J. Quant. Elect.* 9, 992 (1973); J. B.
    Trenholme, et al., to be published in *IEEE J. Quant.
    Elect.;* P. C. Magnante, *IEEE J. Quant. Elect.* 8, 440
    (1972).

20. Some recent publications on CO short-pulse amplifiers
    are: J. L. Lachambre, et al., *IEEE J. Quant. Elect.*
    9, 459 (1973); T. F. Stratton, et al., *ibid* 9, 157
    (1973); M. C. Richardson, et al., *ibid* 9, 236 (1973);
    F. Rheault, et al., *Opt. Commun.* 8, 132 (1973).

21. Iodine laser design and performance are discussed by
    K. Hohla and K. L. Kompa, *Z. Naturforsch.* 27A, 938
    (1972); *Appl. Phys. Lett.* 22, 77 (1972); 18, 48 (1971).

22. C. G. Freeman, et al., *Chem. Phys. Lett.* 6, 482
    (1970); R. H. Newman, et al., *Trans. Far. Soc.* 67,
    2827 (1970); O. P. Strausz, et al., *J. Am. Chem.
    Soc.* 95, 732 (1973).

23. M. A. Gusinow, J. K. Rice, and T. D. Padrick, *Chem.
    Phys. Lett.* 21, 197 (1973).

24. R. M. Hill, D. J. Eckstrom, D. C. Lorents and H. H.
    Nakano, *Appl. Phys. Lett.* 23, 373 (1973).

25. E. E. Huber, D. A. Emmons, and R. M. Lerner, MIT
    Lincoln Laboratory Report JA 4236 (1973); J. Jortner,
    et al., *J. Chem. Phys.* 42, 4250 (1965).

26. Xe_2^* Laser: N. G. Basov, V. A. Danilychev, and Yu. M.
    Popov, *Sov. J. Quant. Elect.* 1, 18 (1971); H. A.

Koehler, L. J. Ferderber, D. L. Redhead, P. J. Ebert, *Appl. Phys. Lett.* <u>21</u>, 198 (1972); P. W. Hoff, J. C. Swingle, and C. K. Rhodes, *Opt. Commun.* <u>8</u>, 128 (1973); E. R. Ault, et al., *IEEE J. Quant. Elect.* <u>9</u>, 1031 (1973); J. B. Gerardo and A. W. Johnson, *J. Appl. Phys.* <u>44</u>, 4120 (1973); E. V. George and C. K. Rhodes, *Appl. Phys. Lett.* <u>23</u>, 139 (1973). Kr_2^* Laser and Ar-Xe Transfer Laser: P. W. Hoff, J. C. Swingle, and C. K. Rhodes, *Appl. Phys. Lett.* <u>23</u>, 139 (1973). Ar-Xe Transfer Kinetics: A. Gedanken, J. Jortner, B. Raz, and A. Szöke, *J. Chem. Phys.* <u>57</u>, 3456 (1972).

27. R. S. Mulliken, *J. Chem. Phys.* <u>52</u>, 5170 (1970).

28. A recent discussion with a bibliography is found in S. Penzes, H. S. Sandlin, and O. P. Strausz, *Int. J. Chem. Kinet.* <u>4</u>, 449 (1972).

29. J. C. W. Johns, *J. Mol. Spectrosc.* <u>36</u>, 488 (1970).

30. C. D. Cooper, G. C. Cobb, and E. L. Tolnas, *J. Mol. Spectrosc.* <u>7</u>, 223 (1961).

31. C. A. Slocomb, W. H. Miller, and H. F. Schaefer III, *J. Chem. Phys.* <u>55</u>, 926 (1971); V. Bondbey, P. K. Pearson, and H. F. Schaefer III, *J. Chem. Phys.* <u>57</u>, 1123 (1972); W. E. Baylis, *J. Chem. Phys.* <u>51</u>, 2665 (1969); A. V. Phelps, *J.I.L.A.* Report #110, University of Colorado, 1972.

32. A. C. Vikis and D. J. Leroy, *PHys. Lett.* <u>44A</u>, 325 (1973); J. B. West, *J. Chem. Phys.* <u>58</u>, 5844 (1973).

33. B. Brocklehurst, *Trans. Far. Soc.* <u>63</u>, 274 (1966); E. Kugler, *Ann. Physik (7)* <u>14</u>, 137 (1964).

34. This possible laser is discussed in more detail by J. R. Murray and C. K. Rhodes, Lawrence Livermore Report UCRL 51455 (1973). Available from NTIS.

35. *Physics of the Aurora and Airglow*, J. W. Chamberlain, Academic Press, New York (1961).

36. Rate constants are from R. J. Donovan and D. Husain, *Chem. Rev.* 70, 489 (1970); A. Corney and O. M. Williams, *J. Phys.* B5, 686 (1972); W. Felder and R. A. Young, *J. Chem. Phys.* 56, 6028 (1972); and from D. Garvin, U. S. Dept. of Commerce, NBS Report NBSIR 73-206 (1973).

37. M. Huber, *Phys. Lett.* 12, 102 (1964); H. P. Broida and E. Miescher, *IEEE J. Quant. Elect.* 9, 1629 (1973).

38. M. Zelikoff, K. Watanabe, and E. C. Y. Inn, *J. Chem. Phys.* 21, 1643 (1953).

39. R. A. Young, G. Black, and T. G. Slanger, *J. Chem. Phys.* 49, 4769 (1968); M. C. Dodge and J. Heicklen, *Int. J. Chem. Kin.* 3, 269 (1971).

40. R. Atkinson and K. H. Welge, *J. Chem. Phys.* 57, 3687 (1972); T. G. Slanger, B. J. Wood, and G. Black, *Chem. Phys. Lett.* 17, 401 (1972).

41. G. M. Lawrence, *J. Chem. Phys.* 57, 5616 (1972).

42. G. W. Taylor and D. W. Setzer, *Chem. Phys. Lett.* 8, 51 (1971); W. L. Starr, *J. Chem. Phys.* 55, 5419 (1971).

43. W. Felder, W. Morrow, and R. A. Young, *Chem. Phys. Lett.* 15, 100 (1972).

44. A. Chutjian, G. A. Segal, and H. S. Taylor, submitted to *J. Chem. Phys.* The reaction is analogous to $N_2(A) + O(^3P)$ which has been studied by J. A. Meyer, et al., *Astrophys. J.* 167, 1023 (1969); K. Henriksen, *Planet. Sp. Sci.* 21, 763 (1973).

45. There are a number of references in *Active Nitrogen*, A. N. Wright and C. A. Winkler, Academic Press, New York (1968); see also J. Noxon, *J. Chem. Phys.* 36, 926 (1962).

46. S. Dondes, P. Harteck, and C. Kunz, *Z. Naturforschung* 19a, 6 (1964); *Rad. Res.* 27, 174 (1966).

46. Stimulated Raman scattering is reviewed by W. Kaiser and M. Meier in Chap. E2 of *Laser Handbook* , ed. by F. T. Arecchi and E. O. Schultz-Dubois, North-Holland, Amsterdam (1972).

48. Related two-quantum transitions (in uninverted media) are discussed by, e.g., P. P. Sorokin and J. R. Lankard, *IEEE J. Quant. Elect.* 9, 227 (1973); N. Tanno, et al., *IEEE J. Quant. Elect.* 9, 423 (1973).

49. E. U. Condon, *Phys. Rev.* 41, 759 (1932).

50. M. E. Crawford and R. E. MacDonald, *Can. J. Phys.* 36, 1022 (1958); H. L. Buijs and H. P. Gush, *Can. J. Phys.* 49, 2366 (1971).

51. D. Vienne, M. C. Bigeon, and J. P. Barrat, *Opt. Commun.* 6, 261 (1972).

52. Resonant Antistokes Raman scattering is reviewed (in a somewhat different context) by Y. S. Bobovich and A. V. Bortkevich, *Sov. Phys. Vspekhi*, 14, 1 (1971).

53. A. V. Vinsgradov and E. A. Yukov, *JETP Lett.* 16, 447 (1972).

54. For a discussion of transient scattering see R. L. Carman, et al., *Phys. Rev.* A2, 60 (1970) and Ref. 47.

55. The geometrical factors involved in the relative cross sections are the same as those calculated by Crawford and MacDonald (Ref. 50).

56. Gain has been demonstrated on this transition (R. Carman and H. Lowdermilk, to be published), since these notes were prepared.

57. A. V. Phelps, *Phys. Rev.* 114, 1071 (1959).

LASER FUSION
Richard Morse

The articles on laser fusion that have appeared in
the literature in the last year or two have been mostly
either detailed scientific journal articles for the expert
or qualitative articles for the layman. A short collection
of the journal references is given below. This lecture
will attempt a compromise in two parts: (I) A long "back
of the envelope" calculation intended to give an audience
of laser specialists a quantitative feeling for the orders
of magnitude involved in the fusion end of a laser fusion,
followed by (II) several short qualitative discussions of
some of the more complex problems glossed over in the
first part.

8.1. FUSION YIELDS AND SCALING

We start out in the first part of this lecture by
considering a fusion target consisting of a frozen ball of
equal number densities of deuterium and tritium. DT is the

favorite thermonuclear fuel because a deuterium-tritium
collision has the largest nuclear fusion cross section at
low energies, i.e., energies corresponding to fuel temperatures of a few tens of keV. We note that the Boltzmann
distribution averaged cross section, which rises rapidly
around 5 keV, begins to roll over near 10 keV. The maximum is at 70 keV, but the curve is very flat there.[1] Not
wishing to invest unnecessary energy in heating the fuel,
we choose 10 keV as an interesting temperature. We will
further assume that electrons as well as ions must be
heated, although electron-ion temperature equilibration
times in some cases are slow enough that this is not
necessary--more about this later.

The energy per ion is then

$$\epsilon = \frac{3}{2} kT \times 2 \text{ (ion and electron)}$$

$$= \frac{3}{2} \times 1.6 \times 10^{-19} \text{ joules/ev} \times 10^{4} \text{ ev} \times 2 \qquad (1)$$

$$= 4.8 \times 10^{-15} \text{ joules/(ion-electron pair)}.$$

The average mass per ion is

$$m = \frac{1}{2} \times (2 + 3) \text{ (AMU)} \times 1.67 \times 10^{-24} \text{ gm/AMU}$$

$$\qquad (2)$$

$$= 4.18 \times 10^{-24} \text{ gm/ion}.$$

We anticipate that an interesting fuel mass will be about
1 μgm and calculate that the number of ions in 1 μgm is

$$N = 10^{-6} \text{ gm} / 4.18 \times 10^{-24} \text{ gm/ion} = 2.4 \times 10^{17} \text{ ions.}$$

$$(3)$$

The total energy invested at 10 keV is then

$$E_{IN} = 2.4 \times 10^{17} \text{ ions} \times 4.8$$

$$\times 10^{-15} \text{ joules/(ion-electron pair)} \qquad (4)$$

$$= 1,150 \text{ joules,}$$

which seems to be a reasonable, perhaps even a modest energy to expect from short pulsed lasers of the near future.
Somewhat larger energies will be required, however, because
of inefficiencies in the heating process. We now ask about
the size of this pellet of fuel, given that it is spherical
and that the normal solid density of DT is

$$\rho_{\text{solid DT}} = 0.213 \text{ gm/cm}^3 . \qquad (5)$$

$$M = 10^{-6} \text{ gm} = \frac{4\pi}{3} \times R^3 \times 0.213 \text{ gm/cm}^3$$

$$= .892 \ R^3 \text{ gm/cm}^3 \quad \text{or} \qquad (6)$$

$$R = 1.04 \times 10^{-2} \text{ cm} = 104 \ \mu\text{m.}$$

For the normal solid salt, L_iDT, $\rho \simeq 1$ gm/cm^3 and
$R \simeq .62 \times 10^{-2}$ cm for a 1 μgm ball.

We will also want the density of ions or electrons in
frozen DT;

$$n_{e,i} = .213 \text{ gm/cm} /4.18 \times 10^{-24} \text{ gm/ion}$$

$$= 5.10 \times 10^{22} \ (e,i/\text{cm}^3).$$

(7)

The plasma pressure of this solid density DT when
heated to a temperature of 10 keV is

$$P = nkT = \frac{2}{3} n\left(\frac{3}{2} kT\right) = \frac{2}{3} \times 5.10 \times 10^{22} \ (e,i/\text{cm}^3)$$

$$\times 4.8 \times 10^{-8} \text{ ergs/}(e,i \text{ pair})$$

(8)

$$= 1.63 \times 10^{15} \text{ dynes/cm}^2 .$$

(While most of us initially have very little feeling for
such pressure units, one quickly learns to think of 10^{15}
as a moderate pressure and of 10^{17} or 10^{18} as a large
pressure).

In order to estimate the characteristic times of
laser fusion events we need the speed of sound. In the
ideal gas approximation the speed of sound depends only on
temperature, and at 10 keV, using P and ρ from above for
simplicity, although $n_{e,i}$ cancels out, and the ideal gas
ratio of specific heats, $\gamma = 5/3$, we obtain

$$C_s = \sqrt{\frac{\gamma P}{\rho}} = \sqrt{\frac{5}{3} \times \frac{1.63 \times 10^{15} \text{ dynes/cm}^2}{.213 \text{ gm/cm}^3}}$$

(9)

$$= 1.13 \times 10^8 \text{ cm/sec}.$$

This is slightly faster than a 10 keV deuteron.

Suppose now that the pellet is heated uniformly to
a temperature of 10 keV before it can expand significantly.
This supposition implies that thermal conduction is sufficiently large to permit laser pulse energy absorbed at
the surface of the pellet to be conducted into the pellet
in the time allowed and that sufficiently intense and rapidly rising laser pulses can be generated and focused to
give the desired heating in the time allowed. Also since
electron thermal conduction is in general larger than that
of ions, but it is the ion temperature which leads to fusion, we are implicitly making some assumptions about
electron-ion thermal equilibration rates. There are
reservations and clarifications that go with all of these
assumptions, some of which are discussed in Part II, but if
these were impossibly restrictive this lecture would not
have been given.

We then ask how long it takes our uniform sphere of
10 keV DT plasma to disassemble. The mode of disassembly
of such a pressurized fluid (mean free paths are sufficiently short to justify the use of a fluid description) is
by propagation of a rarefaction wave inward from the surface of the sphere at the speed of sound. Before this
rarefaction arrives at a given interior point, that point
doesn't know that the surface is free to expand, if thermal

conduction can be neglected. Thermal conduction can cool
the center of the plasma ahead of the rarefaction because
the outer part of the plasma that has already expanded has
been cooled by that expansion. However, more detailed calculations show that, while this cooling can be significant,
it does not dominate the results, and, therefore, that it
is useful to calculate the time interval required by a simple adiabatic rarefaction wave to go from the surface of
the sphere to the center;

$$\Delta t = R/C_s = 1.04 \times 10^{-2} \text{ cm}/1.13 \times 10^8 \text{ cm/sec}$$

$$\text{(10)}$$

$$= 92.0 \times 10^{-12} \text{ sec.}$$

It is clear from this that, if laser fusion were to be
approached in this way, the laser pulse length would have
to be of the order of or less than 92 picosec for the target we have chosen. If the pulse length is the Δt above,
then the average laser power is

$$W_L = E/\Delta t = 1{,}150 \text{ joules}/92.0 \times 10^{-12} \text{ sec}$$

$$= 1.25 \times 10^{13} \text{ watts} \qquad \text{(11)}$$

$$= 12.5 \text{ joules/picosec.}$$

This is about one order of magnitude larger than
peak power from present short pulse Nd glass lasers, but
about the design goal of the larger glass and CO_2 systems
now being built.

The rate of thermonuclear fusion burning of D and
T ions at a point in our pellet before the arrival of the
rarefaction is

$$R_{DT} \text{(reactions per } cm^3/\text{sec)} = n_D n_T \langle \sigma v \rangle_{DT} , \qquad (12)$$

where the average of cross section times relative velocity
is an average over a Boltzmann velocity distribution. At
a 10 keV temperature[1]

$$\langle \sigma v \rangle_{DT \text{ @ 10 keV}} \simeq 1.2 \times 10^{-16} \ cm^3/\text{sec} , \qquad (13)$$

and therefore

$$R_{DT} = \left(\frac{1}{2} \times 5.10 \times 10^{22} \ cm^{-3} \right)^2 \times 1.2 \times 10^{-16} \ cm^3/\text{sec}$$

$$= 7.80 \times 10^{28}/cm^3/\text{sec}.$$

The burn power density is calculated with a value of 18×10^6 ev for the DT reaction energy plus a small increment
from a neutron induced breeding reaction in the reactor
wall, which gives

$$W_B = R_{DT} \times 18 \times 10^6 \ ev \times k \times volume$$

$$= 7.80 \times 10^{28}/cm^3/\text{sec} \times 18 \times 10^6 \ ev$$

$$\times 1.6 \times 10^{-12} \ ergs/ev \times \left(\frac{10^{-6} \ gm}{0.213 \ gm/cm^3} \right)$$

that is,

$$W_B = 1.05 \times 10^{19} \text{ ergs/sec} = 1.05 \times 10^{12} \text{ watts.} \quad (15)$$

We estimate the average burn time to be 1/5 of the rare-faction Δt above because about one half of the fuel mass is in the outer 1/5 of the sphere by radius, and because the burn rate drops so sharply just behind the rarefaction on account of the temperature and density dependences that we can regard the rarefaction front as turning off the burn when it passes a point. We have then

$$E_{out} = W_B \times \Delta t/5 = 1.05 \times 10^{12} \text{ watts}$$

$$\times 92.0 \times 10^{-12} \text{ sec/5} \quad (16)$$

$$= 19.3 \text{ joules.}$$

(Very detailed self-consistent calculations of the fusion yield from our preheated expanding sphere give 22 joules).[2] At about 3.4×10^{11} fusion neutrons/joule of E_{out}, this gives about 7×10^{12} neutrons.

The yield ratio, Y_R, is

$$Y_R = E_{out}/E_{in} = 19.3 \text{ joules}/1{,}150 \text{ joules} = 0.018, \quad (17)$$

which is rather small. Since, according to the prescription followed above, the yield ratio is proportional to the radius, the radius must be 1/0.018 = 55.6 times larger to achieve $Y_R = 1$, or

$$R(Y_R=1) = R(M=10^{-6} \text{ gm})/0.018$$

$$= 1.04 \times 10^{-2} \text{ cm} \times 55.6 = 0.577 \text{ cm}. \qquad (18)$$

Because E_{in} increases in proportion to the mass, and, therefore, R^3,

$$E_{in}(Y_R=1) = (55.6)^3 \times 1{,}150 \text{ joules}$$

$$= 1.98 \times 10^8 \text{ joules}, \qquad (19)$$

which is rather large, especially since this is still only scientific breakeven. Hence, we need another way to improve Y_R. Increasing the temperature much above 10 keV doesn't help because E_{in} increases faster than E_{out}.

The scheme that does help is compressing the pellet. From Eq. (12) the burn rate per ion increases in proportion to the density. On the other hand, as the pellet density is increased at a constant temperature the disassembly per burn time decreases in proportion to the decreasing radius. Hence, for a fixed total pellet mass and initial temperature, Y_R changes according to

$$Y_R \sim \rho R \sim \rho^{2/3} \sim 1/R^2 . \qquad (20)$$

According to this scaling law, the factor of 55.6 needed to bring our 1 μgm pellet to breakeven can be achieved by increasing the initial density by $\times 415$, that is, decreasing the initial radius by $\times 0.134$. The value of ρR required for breakeven is then

$$\rho R \text{ (breakeven)} \simeq 0.12 \text{ gm/cm}^2 . \tag{21}$$

As long as all energy production and loss mechanisms are
two (not three) body processes, Y_R is a function of the
parameter ρR and the initial temperature and does not depend on the pellet mass in any other way. Hence, $\rho R = 0.1$
is approximately equivalent to the Lawson criterion for
magnetic confinement breakeven, $n\tau$ (density × confinement
time) = 10^{14} sec/cm^3.

8.2. TECHNIQUES AND PROBLEMS OF LASER FUSION

Ablation Driven Implosion

        The technique which is expected to give us the fuel
compressions discussed above is spherical implosion driven
by ablation pressure.[3,4] Laser light energy absorbed at
the surface of a pellet heats the surface material, causing
it to blow off, i.e., to ablate, and pushing the inside of
the pellet inward by the recoil, like a rocket engine distributed more or less uniformly over the surface of the
pellet pushing radially inward. The ablation pressure
usually drives a converging shock into the initially cold
material and then further adiabatically compresses the
shocked material to densities larger than those produced
by a simple strong shock. In fact, numerical calculations
have shown that if the laser pulse is shaped to give the
right kind of smoothly rising ablation pressure time history, then compressions to several thousand times the initial density can be obtained. A difficulty to be avoided

is initial heating of the center of the fuel to such high
entropy densities that subsequent adiabatic compression of
the fuel to the necessary densities is impossible. This
can come about either because the initial shock is too
strong or because the laser power input is so high that a
nonlinear thermal conduction wave (electron thermal conductivity is proportional to $T_e^{5/2}$)[5] outruns the compression wave and arrives at the center first. The latter
phenomenon, called "burn thru", is harder to avoid in
small pellets.

Shock Heating and Electron-Ion Equilibration

It is believed that absorbed laser light energy goes
almost entirely into the electrons. Moreover, the larger
electron thermal conduction is expected to transport the
absorbed energy from the surface of the pellet inward to
the ablation front. On the other hand, the viscous heating which occurs in a strong shock front is believed to go
almost entirely into the ions. Therefore, ions can be
heated by thermal equilibration with the electrons or by
shocking. The electron-ion thermal relaxation time is proportional to $\rho T_e^{-3/2}$ and is about 10^{-9} sec in the 10 keV,
solid density DT plasma discussed above.[5] Hence, thermal
relaxation can be rather slow. Two temperature models are
required and care must be taken to give the core of the
pellet its entropy by shocking rather than by electron
thermal conduction because the latter may leave the ions
cold through the subsequent adiabatic compression.

Light Absorption at the Critical Surface

According to electromagnetic wave theory, the laser
light that is incident on the surface of a pellet cannot
penetrate deeper into the pellet than the surface, called
the critical surface, on which the electron plasma frequency, which is proportional to $\sqrt{n_e}$, is equal to the
light frequency. This occurs where $n_e = 10^{21}/cm^3$ for the
1.06 μm wavelength light from Nd laser and where $n_e =
10^{19}/cm^3$ for the 10.6 μm light from CO_2. These are respec-
tively 1/50 and 1/5000 of the density of electrons in solid
density DT given above. Hence, the absorption of infrared
light at the surface of initially solid density targets
must occur in the extreme low density part of the blow-off
cloud. This region can be at a considerable distance from
the pellet, in units of the initial radius, during the latter stages of pellet heating and compression. The classical light absorption mechanism is inverse bremsstrahlung,
i.e., collisional damping of the incident light wave.
However, the inverse bremsstrahlung absorption length,
which increases with increasing temperature, is too long to
account for the almost complete absorption that is seen in
many experiments. That is, one would expect to see much
more reflected light than is actually seen. Presumably,
some collective plasma effect is responsible for this anomalous absorption. It would appear, therefore, that the
same kind of enhanced collective effects which make the
magnetic confinement approach to controlled fusion difficult are a source of help to laser fusion.

Restrictions on Electron Thermal Conductivity

According to the classical theory, electron thermal conductivity is independent of plasma density except for a weak logarithmic factor.[5] However, this theory is based on the first order term in an expansion in powers of a measure of the departure of the electron distribution function from its local thermodynamic equilibrium (Maxwellian) form. There is in fact a limit on the amount of heat flux that electrons at a given density and temperature can carry while satisfying certain conservation requirements and collective plasma stability conditions.

This limit, which is in effect based on higher order corrections to the classical theory, can actually noticeably reduce the effective electron thermal conductivity for the high heat fluxes encountered in some laser fusion experiments and at the low electron densities near the critical surface.[6] As the laser light wavelength becomes longer and the critical density becomes correspondingly smaller, the effect of the flux limit for a given input power density is to force the electron temperature near the critical surface higher while making it more difficult to couple the absorbed laser light energy into the interior of the pellet where it is needed to drive the desired implosion. It appears, at the present, that at typical laser fusion critical surface power densities of a few times 10^{14} w/cm^2 up to 10^{15}, the flux limit at the critical density of 10.6 μm CO_2 light is just at the verge of causing difficulty. However, we believe that we can live with the problem, especially in view of the great advantages of the CO_2 laser over any other high power, short pulse laser system now

available. We must, however, be alert to the possibility
that collective phenomena may limit local departures from
thermodynamic equilibria more severely than we now have any
reason to expect, and make the flux limit problem correspondingly more severe.

Ignition and Propagating Burn

When estimating fusion energy yields above, we
implicitly concentrated on low yield situations up to
breakeven, whereas in fact the real economic interest centers on yield ratios of one hundred or more. When E_{out}
approaches or exceeds E_{in}, the redeposition of fusion
energy into the fuel from reaction products, especially α
particles, can significantly increase the fuel temperature,
and with it the reaction rate. When the fusion energy redeposition rate exceeds the rate of energy loss from
bremsstrahlung (which we have also ignored up to now), a
condition called ignition occurs in which the temperature
and reaction rate can rise very rapidly and the final yield
ratio can be considerably increased. If all the α particles are captured in the fuel and all of the bremsstrahlung is lost, which is a reasonable approximation for many
cases of interest, then the DT ignition temperature is
about 4 keV.[7] A further major improvement in the yield
ratio occurs if as a result of the spherically converging
nature of the implosion only the very center of the fuel
is heated above the ignition temperature while the remainder
of the fuel remains much cooler. If, in addition, the hot
center region has a ρR of one or two or more by itself,
it may not only ignite but, in turn, ignite adjacent cold

fuel through thermal conduction, hydrodynamic expansion
and transport of reaction products.[2] This propagating burn
behavior is responsible, and seemingly necessary for, the
yield ratios of 100 or more that have been obtained from
some pellet implosion and burn calculations.[3,4]

Hollow Shells and Increased Pulse Length

An important point which we glossed over above is
that when pulses are shaped so as to obtain good implosions,
the resulting shape has a long, weak precursor, but the
full-width at half-maximum is in general somewhat less than
we would estimate on acoustic transit arguments (e.g., the
92 picosec estimated above for a 1 μgm sphere of solid DT).
Since shorter high energy pulses are increasingly hard to
generate, we have sought target configurations that can be
successfully ignited with longer and less precisely shaped
pulses.

In Ref. 4 laser driven implosions of hollow shells
of solid DT have been simulated numerically and shown to
work about as well as solid spheres. There a highly shaped
and optimized pulse was used with both spheres and shells.
However, hollow shells are, in a sense, at their best when
the pulse employed is broad and less structured because
they are less sensitive to pulse shape. In particular,
when the pellet radius is increased by making the pellet a
hollow shell, then it takes longer for the pellet to implode at a given inward velocity, and the usable laser
pulse length is correspondingly increased. One cannot go
on indefinitely in this direction, however, because when

the thickness of the shell becomes too much smaller than its radius, it becomes difficult to achieve a sufficiently symmetric implosion with a finite number of laser beams heating the outside of the shell.[8] The author expects that a factor of three increase in usable pulse length can be achieved in this way, but that a factor of ten would be rather difficult, at least until we get to much higher energies and larger pellets where greater precision may be easier to obtain.

REFERENCES

1. J. L. Tuck, *Nucl. Fusion* 1, 202 (1961).

2. G. S. Fraley, E. J. Linnebur, R. J. Mason and R. L. Morse, *Phys. Fluids*, January 1974.

3. J. Nuckolls, L. Wood, A. Thiessen, and G. Zimmerman, *Nature* (London) 239, 139 (1972).

4. J. S. Clarke, H. N. Fisher and R. J. Mason, *Bull. Am. Phys. Soc.* 17, 1035 (1972), *Phys. Rev. Lett.* 30, 89 (1973), and 30, 249 (1973).

5. L. Spitzer, *Physics of Fully Ionized Gases*, Chap. V, Interscience, New York (1969).

6. R. L. Morse and C. W. Nielson, *Phys. Fluids* 16, 909 (1973).

7. S. Glasstone and R. H. Loveberg, *Controlled Thermo-nuclear Reactions*, Van Nostrand, Princeton, New Jersey, (1960), p. 33.

8. D. B. Henderson and R. L. Morse, *Phys. Rev. Lett.* 32, 355 (1974).

INDEX

INDEX